Leathersex
A Guide for the Curious Outsider and the Serious Player

LEATHERSEX

*A Guide
for the Curious Outsider
and the Serious Player*

Joseph W. Bean

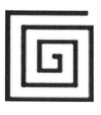 Daedalus Publishing Company

Published by
Daedalus Publishing Company
2140 Hyperion Ave.
Los Angeles, CA 90027
USA
http://www.daedaluspublishing.com

Cover Design by Steve Diet Goedde

Library of Congress Catalog Card Number: 94-71570

ISBN 1-881943-05-4

Printed in the United States of America

I dedicate this book to Scott Smitherum. In the small circle of my life, no one has meant more to me or done more for me than he has. I set this book as a milepost in my battle against his enemies: prudery, homophobia, and AIDS.

ABOUT THE AUTHOR

Joseph W. Bean is working on several leather history book projects. He served as the first Executive Director for the Leather Archives & Museum in Chicago from 1997 until 2002. He has also edited and/or been the managing editor of *Drummer, Mach, Foreskin Quarterly, Sandmutopia Guardian, Bear, Powerplay, Roundup, MastHead, NLA Quarterlink, International Leatherman, Bunkhouse* and many other leather/SM magazines and newsletters. He originated the magazines *Tough Customers* and *Hombres Latinos*. His writing—including books, articles and speeches—are widely read and often cited in educational settings from leatherfests to Universities. He was, for more than 15 years, among the most active speaker-demonstrator-instructors in North American leather, and was a regular guest lecturer and SM demonstrator at San Francisco State University for five years. Perhaps all these years of activity explain why he now lives on Maui, in the middle of the Pacific Ocean, where he settled in 2002.

CONTENTS

Foreword

When I took my tentative first steps into the leather world over 15 years ago, the only things guiding me were lies and myths. Deviant sex is bad. Its practitioners are sick, or worse–evil. Even to admit to masochistic feeling is a sign of unpardonable weakness. It was hard to imagine more fearsome boogiemen at the gates of self-exploration than these.

Yet somehow I managed to get past the totems of taboo and indulge long pent-up desire. Getting there is half the fun, the saying goes, but how much better for me and others if I had been able to count on the type of reliable insight offered in the following pages by Joseph W. Bean.

One of the things I know now that I didn't know then, is that entering the realm of leathersex is really about coming into one of the most vibrant communities of men and women around. It took years before I could trust the integrity of my instincts or be honest about the need locked in my fantasies. Those twin demons of guilt and shame had conspired well to keep me from the celebration I sought. Even more to the point, my repression kept me from knowing others who had explored radical sexuality and had lessons to teach.

That unhappy chapter of my life was closed some time ago, but it has left a lingering resolve to help overcome the fear and loathing society preaches about those who would dare venture beyond its narrow vision. Today, I see leatherfolk as an advance guard pushing on the boundaries of human capacity and understanding. Their tools and techniques are implements for a new kind of spiritual technology. They are wounded healers and crazy ritual makers, astute sexual warriors and funky members of a tribe. But above all, they are people who feel much as I do: that beneath censure and uncertainty there lies a freedom that, for us, can be found best through leathersex.

So what is it, exactly, that we do? Are we sado-masochists, as the clinically minded would avow. Or are we advocates of "sensuality and mutuality" or even "sex magic," as some today are claiming. With candor and wisdom, Bean is able to walk a carefully reasoned line through all the meanings to be found in the experience known as SM; he neither shies away from its earthy realities nor skirts its transcendent possibilities. He's well-grounded in leather's "old guard" sensibility, a semi-mythic world of sexual outlaws and loners meeting tough and fast on the urban fringe, and advances notions from a new wave of leather-clad sensualists who are bringing fresh elements into their play. Most important, Bean provides page after page of clear-headed and practiced advice for those wanting to explore sexual frontiers.

The fact that so much of what is described here has been traditionally forbidden makes *Leathersex* of interest to a wide variety of readers–not just the inquisitive tyro or seasoned practitioner. The hows and whys of the scene–from basic technique to psychological theory–are amply covered, but Bean attempts something else too. He delves deeper than almost any other nonfiction writer on the subject to explore what makes leather–and all that it implies–so alluring and necessary for so many. Sociologists, therapists, and any student of human nature would be better educated about sex and psyche by reading this book.

Above all, Bean teaches honesty. Leathersex is a tempering experience, often providing initiation into aspects of self left untapped or hidden. Through extreme and volatile acts, it can jolt and transport its players to surprising places. In many cases, engaging in leathersex is like dancing on the brink of an abyss. That is its fascination and, also, its danger.

There is no room for subterfuge or secret agendas when two people come together for leathersex. Power is given and taken. Personal identity can be peeled away and put on a shelf. Vulnerabilities are often exposed and primal sides of the soul let loose. Sometimes, sacred inner places are found as well. Bean knows all of these things, but like any competent guide he outlines the highs and lows of the terrain while leaving some spots unmentioned–the better left for one's own careful discovery.

The ability to mediate extremes–in writing as well as life–seems to come naturally to the author. Born in Humansville, Missouri in 1947, Bean began to write for publication and experiment with leathersex at about the same time during his adolescence. "I have tried to walk away from both any number of times," he's remarked, "but have found that I don't like my life without them." Since leaving home, Bean has traveled all over the world, curiosity his ticket.

His spiritual searching has resulted in his teaching at a Tibetan Buddhist institute, being made a sheik of the Mevlevi Dervishes, and following the practices of Russian mystic Gurdjieff. Bean has not neglected the exploration of his erotic self; during one period in the 1960s he danced nude for a living on a Los Angeles stage, modeled for photographers, and made numerous gay films. Along this adventurous route, he plunged further into the leather scene in Europe and North America.

Bean's work as a serious journalist has appeared in a variety of publications during the past 20 years, but it was not until the late 1980s that his spiritual and sexual interests began to find common ground. Prompted by the urging of friends, Bean started to write "Leathersex Fairy," a column of opinion and advice syndicated to gay newspapers across the country. This, in turn, led to a tenure as Editor of *Drummer*, the nation's largest magazine addressing the leather lifestyle. And increasingly he spoke out about leatherfolk and their ways in settings ranging from university classrooms to television.

Finally, in this book, we have the sum of his experience. There are few people as versed about the truths and falsehoods of radical sexuality–and better able to share that information with depth and conviction–than Joseph Bean. He is a dexterous voyager to places both dark and light, sensational and serene. A companionable educator, in the way a good master can be, we are better off for having his knowing hand in *Leathersex*.

Mark Thompson, Editor
The Advocate

Preface

"Prudery kills." Playwright Robert Chesley told me that as his introduction to an interview I did with him in 1988 for *Coming UP!*, a gay/lesbian monthly newspaper in San Francisco. At the end of the interview, when the tape recorder was off, and we were just chatting about the effects of the AIDS epidemic on our lives, he said it again. "Prudery kills, and the more we go around showing ourselves to be sexual, proud and sexual, the greater force we can be to stand against that killer." Two and a half years later, on December 5, 1990, Chesley died. My first thought was, "Prudery kills again." I asked myself then if I was standing as strongly as I could against it. I still don't know if I am doing all I can, but I know this book is a volley that will be at least a little annoyance to some of the soldiers of prudery.

This book, therefore, is a small contribution to what is still the beginning of an exploration I hope will be actively continued. It is a distant cousin, probably a poor relative, of Chesley's plays. It has a very specific point of view—mine—and makes no attempt to be all things to all readers. I am gay, male, middle-aged, white, American, and a romantic. All these things, as well as my sexual history, inform and limit what my book can be. People different from myself in every possible way should examine the truth about radical sexuality in their own lives and communities and share their discoveries. Nearly a century of studies in human sexuality have proven that no scholarly outsider conducting interviews and observations can give us the beating hearts and sweating palms that are essential to a real understanding of what makes sex exciting. I intend to support and encourage all efforts by kinky people of every sort to present themselves and their sexual behaviors honestly. If nothing else, the more of us there are who tell the whole truth about what gets us off, the more discomfort we can cause for the prudes.

This is not an instruction manual for SM novices, although I hope novices and curious outsiders will find some useful instruction here.

It is not a prescription for sexual satisfaction, although it may nudge some people toward admitting that they can have the pleasures they know they want. It is not an explanation of SM or radical sexuality, although it is intended to explain what I know, believe, and have experienced in SM.

Allow me to tell you something about myself which may help you to decide whether this book can have any value for you: I have recently undertaken the mastery of a new slave. The months or years ahead are to be devoted to his training. This means I will guide him into behaviors and states where his service to me provides me with a comfortable, convenient, erotically challenging, and completely satisfying life. He will do anything I ask. He will take care of my home and my body. He will be beaten and tortured. He will provide me with sex, and see that it is emotionally safe and physically easy for me to do whatever I choose, even if that means flogging others or having sex with them. We share the burden of the life we are embarking upon, even if the scales seem very much tipped in my favor. My slave, warren, would not ask for this life if he were not also expecting that his service to me would give him a fulfilling and exciting life.

I am particularly appreciative of the change in my life heralded by warren's arrival because, for over a year now, I have been a slave to this book. I have awakened every morning searching the requirements of the day for moments when I could freely serve the demands of this manuscript. I have looked forward to days off from everything else, not because I would be able to rest, but because I would be available to the beeps and clicks of this book as it put itself together in my computer.

Mission accomplished. The book has trained me well. Now, as I have done before, I will stretch up out of my slavery to share with a new slave what I have learned and become.

My Master–this book–has demanded that I feed him all my thoughts and experiences of radical sex, all my essays and articles, all my lecture notes and class tapes. He has spit back at me every unworthy sentiment and every ill-considered idea. He has required me to reconsider everything, repeatedly, and caused me to demand more of myself than I imagined I could do. It is the nature of a

Master to do that, to push a slave further into himself and faster along in his life than the slave believes possible.

At times I have wanted to run away from my Master, to leave him and let him find another slave with a computer and typing skills–and more determination than I had. That never quite happened because the very friends I might have run to for escape were as much under my Master's spell as I.

Those friends deserve a lot of the credit for this book because they patiently locked me in with my Master again and again, always telling me no one could serve him better. My gratitude to these "cruel" friends knows no bounds: Scott Smitherum, my slaveboy when I started this project; Mark Thompson, my inspiration for this and any number of other writing projects; Gayle Rubin, Beardog Hoffman, Jay Marston, Victoria Baker, Anthony F. DeBlase, Animal J. Smith, Guy Baldwin, and Mark I. Chester who, by example, gave me the courage to believe in my own strength.

Hal Heller, computer genius and magician, saved the book at a crucial moment. John DeCecco and John Elia have (not always knowingly) played many roles in easing me through my need to write this book, and in encouraging me with patience when I thought the need had passed.

In my experience, Larry Townsend created the genre of SM non-fiction, and, very significantly, he showed only a positive interest in my book each time he heard of it. He never knew what a blessing that was to me.

Much of what has taken shape here in book form was originally prepared for newspapers like *The San Francisco Sentinel*, *Philadelphia Gay News*, and *Out Front* (Denver); for magazines like *The Advocate*, *Drummer*, and *The Sandmutopia Guardian*; for lectures at San Francisco State University, QSM, and various clubs and organizations across the country. By asking me to speak or write for them, by presenting me as an expert, and often by inviting me back, the editors, club officers, and professors involved have added immeasurably to this book.

Chapter One

Getting Started in Leathersex

THINKING THROUGH THE REAL POSSIBILITIES

You want to be a leatherman, do you? Bottom? At least to start, right? Think it over carefully. If what you really want is the sort of leathersex fantasy that dreams and hot magazine fiction are made of–hulking muscularity, extreme brutality, intense scenes that leave no mark except in memory–you might be better off leaving your leathersex in the realm of fantasy. There is nothing wrong with that. Close your eyes, breathe in the sweaty smell of your sex partner, pull against the imaginary restraints. Go ahead, enjoy the amplified pleasure that comes from yoking real sexual activity with the heightened sensations of fantasy.

On the other hand, if the fantasies leave you aching inside, and you want something more, something that leaves you tingling inside and out, maybe leathersex–the dynamic of Top and bottom, genuine SM, bondage, or some kind of leather/levi rough sex–is what you are attuned to. No one is going to tell you that it never hurts to try, but maybe that is just what you want.

How to go about trying leathersex safely is another question altogether. Unfortunately, the first answer to that has to be something negative: Do not try to bluff your way into an SM or leather scene. No pretending. About *anything*. Tell the man or men you are with that you are a novice. Tell him (them) what you think you want, and what you are sure you do not want to try. And, do this before it gets to a point that might be embarrassing for you or disappointing for anyone. This sort of conversation in which you spell out your level of experience, your tastes, and your limits is called "negotiation."

Negotiation is one of the three basic elements of communication among leathermen. The others are "networking" and "feedback." All three of these techniques will be discussed and referred to frequently, but later, in this book. In the meantime, you might like to know something about the guys you'll eventually be communicating with, in and out of the playroom.

In the beginning, finding potential partners for leathersex can be a good deal more difficult for most people than finding partners for more common varieties of sex, if only because there are fewer leathermen. How to find partners who are willing to take a turn with a novice is another matter, and it is not as simple as hanging out in a leather bar. First, you should realize that leathermen are just like all other gay men in some ways–many ways. One thing they have in common with their vanilla brothers is that some of them enjoy "breaking cherries," and some of them are turned off by it. You obviously want the former sort.

Another way that the men you find in a leather bar are like the rest of the gay male population is that many of them are less than completely honest. While the leather lifestyle imposes an important sort of honesty on the men who are serious about it– those who are really part of the leather scene–serious leathermen are only a small part of a leather bar's clientele. Many of the men in the bar are not necessarily what they appear to be, or even what they claim to be. In fact, the naked truth is that most of the people dressed in leather, wearing all sorts of leather signalling devices, dropping their voices into bass registers, and claiming to know nothing of opera, ballet, or quiche . . . most of them are fringe dwellers of a sort that leaves them novices for as long as they hang around the leather venues. They never find out what leathersex *really* is, even if they do get into a leathersex scene now and then.

The results of occasional SM encounters are exhilarating or frightening for the fringe dwellers and flat-out disappointing for the leathermen they are with, *if any*. Fortunately, the most likely partner for a hanger-on is another uninitiated hanger-on. It just works out that way. Bluffers link up with bluffers, while most of the serious players see through the games and steer clear. You do not want to get into this cycle of unproductive, unsatisfying, and really dangerous leather-like sexual escapades. It leads nowhere. Worse, it keeps you from ever connecting with the men you *do* want in your life.

Probably the most common meeting ground on which genuine leathermen connect with each other, despite the less than genuine crowd, is the leather bar. So you will want to look into your local leather bar. In the beginning, a man who is curious about leather should go to the leather bars for reasons that have little to do with either sex or SM. Go, especially when there are contests and shows, beer and soda busts, or public events associated with local clubs, to enjoy the atmosphere, to get a close-enough-to-smell view of leathermen and the scene. Go to have a good time, but be very circumspect about going home with a person you meet at a leather bar but otherwise do not know. Later, when you have trained your tastes, your instincts, and your trust-sensitivity, this will change.

If you have not been going to leather bars, you may find them a bit intimidating, but not for long. Go to the bars to get over fearing them. And, go to the bars for these two very good reasons: First, go to get used to the environment and to gain an understanding of the implications of the things associated with leathermen and their home turf. Second, go because you can collect real faces, flesh, and images of all kinds–realistic images, that is–to beef up your fantasies. If a picture (like the ones in a porn magazine) is worth a thousand words, a popular leather bar's patio jammed with men in leather on a Sunday afternoon is worth a million, at least.

It may even be appropriate to go to leather bars, and to wear enough leather to feel comfortable there, even if you have decided that the fantasies of leathersex are enough for you. Of course, this means the serious leathermen in the bar run the risk of noticing and wanting you, then discovering that you are not interested. This will not be a problem–and you will spare the men who approach you the sense of rejection you might otherwise cause them–if you will just be honest and forthcoming about why you are there. Tell them right away that you are not into leathersex, but you enjoy being among leathermen. This way, rather than getting a reputation for being a cock-tease, you will probably end up with a lot of friends and good companions who also enjoy being with you. Besides, this tactic leaves all options open for the future.

Enjoy leather and leathersex, leathermen and leather bars your way, whatever it is. Whether you want fantasy or reality, action or imagination, do what you want to do, not what some fiction writer has suggested or what you have been told is "the way to act."

When and if you decide you do want to get involved in leather-sex, there are two things you will need to get started, and leather is not one of them. They are preparation and opportunity.

Preparation means having a genuine answer to the question "What're you into?" To have an honest answer that is not just "I don't know," you need to be speaking from *some* experience (or careful consideration) and training (or very careful consideration), not just recalling some recent porn publication.

Opportunity means a chance to get it on with other men who share your tastes. And the right opportunities will be ones that increase your experience and training while taking proper consideration of the fact that you are new to the scene. In other words, the opportunities that work will be ones that feed into your preparation; and the preparation that is appropriate will be the kind that improves your opportunities.

Obviously, the perfect preparation and opportunity for a leather-sex life is to meet the man or men who exactly match your interests, and have him/them experiment with and train you up to the point where both of you are getting exactly what you want out of your sex lives. Failing that–and we do want to be realistic here–one safe, sane, accessible alternative is to find formal training from experienced leathermen and to let the opportunities develop around that.

Formal training sounds a bit strange when the subject is sex. After all, no one has to be taught in a formal way to fuck and suck. Leathersex involves a great deal more, though, including the potential for serious injury, psychological trauma, and even death. And, proving the old saying that necessity is the father of invention, the training that is required is available.

There are a number of well-established groups scattered around the country whose purpose is to provide people interested in leathersex "with a forum in which to share practical information, ideas, feelings, health and safety tips, etc., in a supportive and unloaded atmosphere." Continuing to quote from a Society of Janus handout: "Janus is a vehicle to educate the general public about S/M, and the S/M community about itself." There are chapters of the Society of Janus (under various names, of late) in several West Coast cities. Similar groups have formed over the past ten or more years in most major cities. Where there are no groups formed specifically for SM education and information exchange, one or more local leather/SM clubs is likely to have an instructional outreach program. Hellfire Club, one of the world's most famous SM clubs, has classes in Chicago called "SMU" and Gay Male SM Activists (GMSMA) has educational programs in New York City. Groups like these are the place to go for the kind of information that will lead you to a realistic idea of who you are in relation to leathersex and who the appropriate partners for you are.

SM educators are often far from public. In fact, finding them can be very difficult in some cities. If you go to stores that sell the kinds of clothing and toys leathermen buy, to leather bars, or to events promoted to the leather community, you are likely either to find posters and flyers about the educational possibilities you want, or men who know and will tell you about them. Some of the groups doing instructional programs, like the Brotherhood of Pain in Texas, are for men only. Others, like the Outcasts in San Francisco, are for women only.

The larger the city, the more likely that there will be separate clubs or organizations serving segments of the SM community based on sex, sexual orientation, spiritual interests, level of experience, and so on. Most SM education, however, is offered by groups that have students and members who are male and female; straight, gay, bi, and exploring. The addresses of many organizations that offer some sort of leathersex training are found in magazines like *Drummer* and *The Leather Journal*.

While you are looking up the addresses of local clubs and organizations in leather-related magazines, read the rest of the publication. Look at the ads for products and services, examine the classified and personal ads. Read the club news and commentaries. Give special attention to any how-to articles or other nonfiction published in leathersex magazines. And, read the fiction carefully, considering as you read whether you believe the action described is probably possible or purely fantastic. Then think about what you find in print about the lifestyle you are considering: If life in leather is as much like what is described in leather magazines as life in business is like what business magazines describe, does it still interest you?

Reading magazines, including the fiction in magazines, is a sort of preparation, but be warned that acting out the stories in magazines–although sometimes possible, even sometimes fun–is not the same thing as having a leathersex life of your own. And, while reading magazines is a useful part of preparation, it offers relatively little in terms of opportunity.

It is possible to find people who share your interests in the personal ads in a magazine, but they are not people within the safety of your network. It is possible that an advertisement for a bar or event will interest you, leading eventually to connections and opportunities. But, for the most part, what you want from magazines and other published sources in the way of opportunity is to find the names and addresses of clubs and organizations where you can meet people and safely explore your leathersex interests.

As is so often the case when looking into anything surrounding leather (or any far-from-mainstream lifestyle), caution is the key, even when approaching clubs and organizations. You want to be careful that the group really exists, as opposed to being little more than a club name as a front for someone's personal pleasures. You want to be sure you are given the time–and that you take the time–to get to know the club or organization before you have to make any commitment to it. The most responsible groups will in fact insist that you do this. And, you want to *choose* with whom to associate, rather than sighing and accepting inappropriate associates on the basis of the impression that there is no one else to choose.

A lot of clubs, including many bike clubs, might be relatively sure ways of meeting people and working up to a leathersex experience with them. On the other hand, neither all bike clubs nor all leather clubs are supportive of SM. Having been mistaken so often for leathersex/SM/kinky people, many members of non-SM bike clubs and leather associations have become openly hostile to people who are interested in leathersex. The interests of these bike clubs and leather groups lie in another area. Understand that no matter how much they may look like the men you want to connect with, they are not the individuals who are going to make up your leathersex network.

Similarly, many bathhouses, sex party venues, and producers of sex-permitted events often are, to put it mildly, not entirely welcoming of leathersex in their spaces or at their parties. Sex opportunities in commercial settings, in fact, are very frequently promoted by the use of leather imagery, even though leathersex (beyond a little abusive talk) is seldom encouraged and often not tolerated. Other established sex-palace type businesses and clubhouses are set up for and accepting of only a specific kind of leathersex. Whether the intended action is spanking or fisting, bondage or foot fetishism, these clubs and businesses can be very intolerant of other variants. The reasons for these limiting policies do make sense once you become accustomed to the entire experience the clubs are providing.

The members of these various bike and leather clubs, and the patrons of these sex clubs and special interest sex venues, are not necessarily people to be avoided. There is nothing inherently wrong with *not* being active in leathersex and, consequently, not encouraging it. It is just a matter of being aware of where you are, what is acceptable, and what you may expect.

Still, there are clubs that are very appropriate for leathersex novices. If you feel you are committed to leathersex as a significant part of your lifestyle, you will find a lot of SM clubs very willing to accommodate your inexperience. The best of these, for a novice, are the ones that offer a full range of social and sexual activities. The very best of them will have a system by which interested novices can meet with and talk to a member to ask about the club, the opportunities it offers, and the way a novice should or may approach its members and its functions. The 15 Association in San Francisco, Hellfire Club in Chicago, GMSMA in New York, The Brotherhood of Pain in Houston, and many other SM clubs around the country have among their most prominent members people who are very realistic about the needs of novices, but you must never presume upon your novice condition, never use it as a cover for getting laid by the membership secretary for instance. This is simply the wrong approach, one that is sure to have continuing and unfortunate repercussions.

Many of the better SM/leathersex/kinky clubs in this country and around the world are based on the model of Chicago Hellfire Club. Men from all over the world become familiar with Hellfire and its ways of doing business by attending Inferno, "the annual convention of SM action," and they take the inspiration home to form clubs in their local areas, often without giving credit to Hellfire or calling on the Chicago club for details that are not absorbed in Inferno-only contact with the organization.

The 15 Association in San Francisco, one of the clubs that recognizes and publishes its debt of information and inspiration to Chicago Hellfire Club, says it was established in 1980 "by a group of gay men to promote the *practice* of safe, responsible, consenting sadomasochism (SM), to provide an environment for learning and sharing technique, and to affirm SM as a valid and fulfilling sexual alternative." This group and others like it intend to provide sexual opportunities to "men who have made the decision to be involved in SM and want to expand their horizons, to deepen their knowledge, and to open new contacts and commitments with men into SM."

When you find a club in your area that is sex-positive and leathersex-supportive, it may be one that can be reached only by mail. If this is the case, write, stating your interests fully and carefully in your letter–newsletter, videos, possible future membership, meeting someone to talk to, or whatever–and be sure to make it clear that you are new to the scene.

Clubs pop up sometimes that are formed by novices in the hope of attracting the attention of experienced players. This is not necessarily a bad thing, but it may also not be an answer to your needs. One of the things you are connecting with when you get in touch with an established club is a system of men who have experience and, on that basis, monitor and judge one another constantly. This should not replace your personal judgments and assessments, but it can certainly help by providing a sound foundation of men who are very likely to be trustworthy.

What you can expect from a good leather-brotherhood club is *opportunity*, the opportunity to engage in safe, sane, consensual leathersex in the presence of experienced, concerned, and vigilant club members. Opportunity is the chance, in both social and sexual settings, to meet people who share your interest in leathersex. And, more opportunity is the possibility of relaxing enough (because the setting is safe) to allow yourself to try what you believe you want, to expand your limits within the areas you already know, and to learn about the finer points of leathersex by experience and by association with experienced people. Clubs are not everywhere. Nor are clubs everything. There have to be other opportunities. One obvious option is cruising in bars and other public places, but it circumvents the idea of a network of safe people. Still, if what you want is not going to involve getting yourself restrained in such a way that you might be unable to stop the scene if it goes in a direction you do not want, cruising may be an option for you, even in the beginning. It is most safe if you are a good talker, a good listener, and a good judge of character, but it is not advisable anyway–not for novices.

NETWORKING

To get started, even in an out-of-the-way community where you feel you are "the only one," you should make every effort to develop a reliable network. Even if you have already gotten a start by cruising bars, you probably are not getting to know the men you play with all that well, not building your network of mutually trusted men.

Sometimes, even with the best experiences from pick-ups and tricks, you also get tired of "the hunt," the constant need to search out, attract, work things through with, and then *to trust* a new potential leathersex partner. That can be exhausting in a way that makes leathersex less attractive without decreasing your "need" for it. The most difficult part of it all is the matter of developing trust on little more than eye contact, trusting that what you surmise in a few minutes of bar talk really represents what you can expect in the end. (The pun is all yours.)

There really are better ways to go about it, but for many people– especially novices who have managed to get some early experience by cruising–it will require some lifestyle changes. If your leather life is all in the bedroom, playroom, blackroom, backroom, dungeon, or wherever you have sex, you are in trouble. First, you are missing out on a lot of the pleasures of the leather lifestyles. But the main problem with a sex-only leathersex orientation is that you have no network. You lack the most basic resource you can have for achieving *safely* the satisfaction your sexuality requires.

Leathersex in a blissfully unwedded state relies on the inter-change of the three "ins" among friends: information, introduc-tions, and invitations.

On the information side of the triangle, you need to be hearing who's safe, who's "for real," and who cannot be trusted, especially in scenes involving restraints, actual bondage, or any limitation of your ability to "re-shape" a scene or escape it. You need to be able to find out about sex options that interest you so you aren't unduly surprised if and when you get a chance to try them, and so you can make an informed decision about whether you want to try them. You need to be able to share your discoveries and your excitement with someone who, at least in some overlapping way, shares your interests. And, you need to have a social circle in which you can be your best leather self, if only to insure that you will be able to decently control your conversation in the context of a the sex play scene.

As for introductions, the important factor isn't getting introduced per se. It is being known–really being known–by other men who might introduce you to still other men. And it is knowing the men who might make these introductions, really knowing them. If you and the leathermen you network with know each other well enough, the introductions will make sense. They will be genuine and reason-able responses to who you are and how you want to conduct your social and sexual life.

Of course you'll want to meet the friends of your friends. You'll also meet their tricks and affairs. But the issue of a knowledgeable network of closely associated leather brothers comes to the fore when sex is implied or intended by the introduction, or even when it is a less-than-obvious option. So, you have to be honest with your friends. You must not let the leathermen you associate with be misinformed about your sexual tastes and proclivities, your experi-ence and expertise, or your willingness to experiment.

Then, as much as it may seem on the surface to be an almost irrelevant issue, the last of the three ins is at least as important as the others. It may be the most important. By having a network of friends in leather, you will be sure to be invited to beer busts and other public events, to private social parties, and to sex play parties.

At public events attended with friends and at social parties, you will get to know people you have already met, and you will constantly meet new people who share something of your interest in leather. Ask people about their experience and their acquaintance with other men you know. If you're tactful at all, this will be completely acceptable. Other leathermen will understand that you are checking for your own safety and in the hopes, perhaps, of some future pleasure. They will be doing the same thing. You want to know about the people you are talking to and about the others they know in the local network. And, when you know, from experience, that someone is or isn't into something, that someone is or isn't trustworthy, you will be expected to speak frankly about this. Your safety and that of your friends, new and established, depends on it. (On the other hand, bitchy gossiping is never appreciated!)

At leathersex play parties, you can see for yourself the tastes, habits, and fetishes of other men, and aspects of their trustworthiness–not to mention their organic and "store-bought" equipment. If you are so inclined, you may get to try out sex acts and sex partners in a friendly environment before you try them out in the privacy of your own (or his) dungeon.

All in all, networking is better than cruising as a way to get laid in any leather circle. It is better than picking up strangers as a way of assuring safety in the sex place. By definition, it involves the pleasure of developing friendships among people you have something rather special in common with.

The eventual effect of a healthy network of friends in leather is a safe, sane, and sexually fulfilled leather life. And no one can say they live under conditions that make networking impossible. Even if you live in Eggbert, Alaska, 1,000 miles from the nearest city, you can develop a network by mail, starting from contacts with SM clubs, classified advertisers, leather suppliers, and others. Work at your network as though your life depended on it. It may.

NEGOTIATING

The importance of negotiating with potential play partners once you meet them within your network cannot be overstated. Leathersex offers a seemingly endless array of possible sex acts, and no one likes them all. So, if there were no other reason for it, leathermen would have to negotiate the simple basics of what was to be done by whom to whom and in what order. There is, after all, everything from the usual French and Greek action with a leather overtone to golden showers, scat, bondage, mummification, flogging, shaving, and even permanent body modifications like piercing, tattooing, and scarification. With all that included in the possibilities suggested when two leathermen meet, and a great deal more besides, is it any wonder we have to talk before we get down to the serious business of providing one another with pleasure and pain?

Some scenes can be fairly well advertised with hankies and such. You probably know at least some part of the supposedly universal code: Right for bottoms, left for Tops; yellow for piss, red for fisting, brown for scat, and so on. There are colors for a lot of things, but not everything, and the colors are not universally the same anyway, especially when more exotic tastes are considered. Besides, there are questions of *how* you want to arrive at the advertised sex act, and of how much pain, verbal interaction, or foreplay is right for you. So, hankies aside (on either side), it is always appropriate to talk first and fuck later. Always? Well, no, but you'll know the exceptions when they come up. Just don't get stupid about it.

The talking we're talking about can mean two rather different things. First, it can mean just checking to see if you and the man in front of you are a natural leathersex match. The more off-center your tastes, the less likely this becomes. Second, talking to a potential sex partner can go beyond the question "What're you into?" Then it becomes negotiating in an obvious sense that puts no strain whatever on the usual meaning of the word.

There is no point in trying to negotiate a happy sexual encounter if, for instance, you *must* be fisted and he is repelled by the idea. On the other hand, if you find some areas of mutual and complementary sexual interest, the things you don't naturally agree on may be negotiable.

Suppose you and the man who has caught your eye agree that you should be spanked and forced to suck him off, but you'd also like to service his boots and he'd also like to flog you with a cat-o'-nine-tails. Boot service holds no interest for him, and that cat frightens you. This doesn't have to be the end of the possible meeting. Maybe one of you can give up one of your choice activities, just for the night, just for the sake of getting the rest of your tastes satisfied by someone you have found interesting. Maybe you can let him threaten you with his cat-o'-nine and even drag its knotted thongs across your back between spankings. Maybe he'll let you service his boots if you do it while they're off his feet, or if you can let him force you to do it as punishment for less than perfect oral service.

What it comes down to is this: If you really want this man and he really wants you, something can be worked out. Probably.

Still, you don't want to negotiate yourself into making promises you won't keep, or accepting assurances you don't believe. Nor can you let your groin get ahead of your brain by planting a tricky "maybe" here and an insincere "we'll see" there. If you do this, you'll almost surely be leaving yourself open to some unpleasant surprises, one way and another.

Honesty, clarity, and a willingness to move a little beyond or stop a little short of your ideal sexual encounter can mean everything. It might even mean the night of your life, or possibly stepping slightly sideward into the relationship you didn't even know was possible. If nothing else, giving yourself a little freedom in negotiating sex will lead you to sample new things, to extend your limits in various directions, and to discover sexual possibilities you don't already know in yourself. It will also confirm (or disprove) with controlled experience the distastes you believe yourself to have.

The idea of negotiating sex sounds awful. It sounds so calculating, so unspontaneous. Well, frankly, it is calculating and it is entirely unspontaneous. That is exactly why you want to get it out of the way before anything sexual actually starts to happen. That's not quite true, or not always true. Sometimes the act of negotiating becomes very sexual foreplay. It can even be a way of exploring pretty deeply into fantasy territories you may never actually enter physically. In fact, negotiating can be the beginning of the scene, escalating from "So, you want to do . . . " to "You're going to have to do . . . , if you're ever going to get . . . ," and so on. And it can be hotter than any video or audio tape on the market, being "real" as it is.

For instance, he says he is into humiliation, into humiliating his partner, that is. You have already said you are into piss. In the midst of negotiating the scene you are both hoping will take shape later and elsewhere, he orders you to piss in your jeans. If you do, you have taken a giant step toward saying yes to the man without making any commitment that might have overstepped the currently safe level of the negotiations. What is more, you have already begun to respond to him in a way the two of you have already defined as sexual. It is sex. It is sex in public. It is humiliation, pleasing him (and maybe you). And it is piss, pleasing you (and maybe him).

Another aspect of negotiating the sexual menu with your partner is that it gives you time to size him up in every possible way. You can take a good look into his eyes, and get a real gut-reaction about trusting him, for instance. You can get a reading about mutual honesty, and degrees of seriousness and/or playfulness. In short, negotiating sex can give you time to figure out how to also make the most of it for yourself and your partner.

FEEDBACK

After genuine networking or a careful "hunt" and realistic negotiation, the third element of communication in leathersex is feedback. There is nothing mysterious about this; everyone does it in all kinds of sexual and social situations all the time. It just means letting the man or men you are with know how the action feels to you and whether it is remaining within the range of things you want to accept. The difference between ordinary social or sexual feedback and the feedback required in leathersex is obvious: people get away with lying all the time in everyday situations, including sex, but any dishonesty in a leather scene can be dangerous.

The power exchange, the flow of energy between two people in a leathersex scene, can sometimes allow an intensity of pain or an act for which the bottom is unprepared. A right-headed bottom will not just start shrieking to end the scene in this case, but will want to see the scene adjusted to conform to his limits. A right-headed Top will have provided the means by which this can be done. The usual way of stopping actions or pains that are unbearable or unacceptable is a "safe word."

While safe words have many names, they always serve the same purpose: they assure the bottom of the possibility of stopping the action if it becomes necessary to do so. Whether they are called safe words, exit words, stops, resists, panic buttons, or some other thing, they are (1) agreed upon by both parties, (2) used by the bottom, and (3) *never* ignored.

We will call the device we are talking about a safe word. For example, you might agree with your partner that, if you cannot go on for whatever reason, you will simply say, "Please, halt, Sir." This phrase is a particularly good safe word because it retains the sense of the scene in the words "please" and "Sir," and communicates the urgency of the moment with "halt," a word no bottom should ever utter except in extreme circumstances.

The idea here is not to have to bail out of the scene altogether just because a restraint is too tight or a flogging has become a bit too intense, but to have a negotiated and accepted way of stopping *for the moment*. A part of the agreement is usually that, in the event the safe word is used, the Top will find out what the problem is before he breaks the character and flow of the scene. It may be that the bottom has surprised himself by getting into some sort of panic state that really requires a few minutes' rest from the scene. It may be that the negotiated limits have been passed, or that the bottom is discovering he can bear less than he thought.

Whatever the case, the safe word should not be spoken unless it is entirely necessary, nor should the speaking of the safe word destroy the scene for either party. Shouting for the Top to stop, when a safe word has not been set, could just seem like part of the scene, a hot urging rather than a problem. On the other hand, using the safe word for tiny discomforts that you could have withstood will surely undermine and sour the power exchange.

Many people, especially seasoned players, choose to have two or even three levels of safe words. And, in some cases, another word is agreed upon which is meant to be a go-ahead spoken by the bottom to the Top when the Top questions whether all is well. This latter, extra word is usually superfluous, and often destructive of the mental part of the scene, but it might be useful for bottoms doubtful about their own tastes, interests, and limits.

The two or three levels of safe words are assigned meaning in the course of negotiating the scene. Often, the first word means something like, "Please, Sir, check on the details of the scene as it is at this time because something is not working for me." This level of response should be used early enough in any problem situation to leave it up to the Top to respond appropriately or decide not to respond. Frequently, a good Top will answer the first-level safe word by working the response into the scene in such a way that there is no obvious reaction, but the problem is resolved anyway.

The second-level safe word means that something must be fixed or changed if we are to go on. Or, put another way, "Sir, everything must stop for a while, perhaps until I recover from the problem that is being resolved here, but let us be prepared to continue when I can." This word, for instance, would be used if the bottom feels that his restraints are dangerously pinching nerves or blood vessels, or the action is moving too fast. As with the first-level safe word, this one can often be answered without disturbing the scene. "I'm going to let you have your hands free for a few minutes, slave, while I get myself a cigarette, but don't you dare move."

The third-level safe word, when used to its best advantage, indicates that something is terribly wrong and that the scene should be stopped, probably completely stopped, likely not to be resumed in the next several minutes or hours. This one might translate to something like, "Stop now. Stop it all. It isn't working for me and/or you are not doing what we agreed was acceptable. Let me go *now!*"

There are definitely limits on what a safe word can be. It must never be something that you might say incidentally in a scene. Some bottoms, for example, moan such things as "I can't take it" or "No, please, Sir, stop," meaning that it is all too lovely and perfect and delicious and that they would, if they could, have it go on forever just as it is. Such bottoms should never agree to safe words that include "I can't," or "stop," or "no." A good safe word is one that you cannot forget, that you would never speak without thinking of the need for it, and that you are sure will be clearly understood when spoken.

Who says "halt" these days? Who says "enough" in a scene? Who says "hold off" in any situation? These are good safe words because they are not going to be said unintentionally, nor are they going to destroy the nature of the scene, especially if coupled with a proper tone of voice and some other words like "please" and "Sir."

By agreeing on a safe word, you will find yourself able to agree also on more complete restraint, more intense pain, and more satisfying submission. And you will be able to communicate your need to have a particular activity eased up or stopped without sacrificing what remains of the scene.

A Top who cannot tolerate a safe word–and there are such people–is not a good option for you in the first years of your leathersex experience, and maybe never. A good Top, in fact, will insist on a safe word, will order you to memorize one, and will probably force you to rehearse it so that he has heard what it sounds like coming from you. With the safe word in place, the trust the Top expects is more easily arrived at, and the nerves of the novice bottom are more likely to be at peace.

Some variations on the safe word are useful too. For instance, some Tops don't want the bottom to speak at all, or they want the bottom gagged. In such cases, it can be enough of a safe "word" in some situations to look at the Top's face or into his eyes. If you are not restrained or bound, a hand gesture can be agreed upon, often something as simple as placing the hands in a flat, praying position. Fists are not a good safe-word replacement. They can be made involuntarily while you, as the bottom, are still perfectly willing to have the scene go on.

Safe words are not the only feedback in a leathersex scene. Good Tops can usually read the body language, physiological responses, and changing attitude of a bottom very accurately as well. The back that is being beaten may push and spread, inviting the whip, or it may flinch and draw away. Only experience will give the Top a clear reading of exactly what means what, but the superficial suggestions are fairly obvious. Muscles that are not being stimulated may begin to register reactions, breathing will change, and the volume and type of sound the bottom is making will also vary. These and many other signals from the bottom are involuntary, usually even unconscious, communications. Good Tops see and hear all of it, responding to anything that has real significance by continuing, accelerating, slowing down, or completely changing the action.

Out of these things–networking, negotiation, and feedback–comes the possibility of safe and interesting scenes and satisfying leathersex. A person who has a grasp of these things has the key to managing safely in SM from the very beginning.

TAKING ACTION

Did you ever lower yourself, one timid body part at a time, into a tub of steaming water, only to discover that the water wasn't *that* hot after all. Maybe you even had to add more hot water after you were in, just to get really comfortable. Getting into the leather scene, especially into the public leather scene–meaning bars rather than clubs–is like that. There's a smoke screen of rumors, fantasies, and misunderstandings. There's a certain steam rising off a guy's own feelings about his potential inadequacy or other doubts about himself. And there is always the simple apprehension that comes from facing the unfamiliar.

How to get into the leather scene? Just go for it. One timid body part at a time is okay, but start with your head. That means understanding, for example, that a bar is a bar and a man is a man . . . and cruising, of course, is cruising. There are differences between leather bars, leathermen, leather cruising, and all their non-leather counterparts, but you will learn them quickly if you have your "head in the right space" to begin with.

Here are the head rules. They are all based on generalities about leathermen, and generalities are generally faulty. Nonetheless, we have to start somewhere.

Rule One: Understand that leathermen have explored and gone beyond the personal ground of accepting their homosexuality. Besides coming out, if only to themselves, as gay men they have taken an additional step of coming out as gay *leather*men. In fact, everything about the leathersex lifestyles celebrates and affirms sexuality. Moving into this territory is a major step and it creates a certain confidence in the people who make it consciously. This confidence–both the real thing and the overacted sham you'll see in some leathersex circles–can be intimidating. Don't worry. It's part of the steam rising off the scene.

Rule Two: Be prepared to be honest. Serious leathermen trade in honesty, which is possibly a by-product of that second coming out. For all the fantasies and images, all the shifting of desires and telling of tall tales, the big-T truth is an essential element of safe leather sexuality. If you have to lie–especially about your sexual desires or sexual history–or you doubt that you can distinguish between mental foreplay and lying, hang back. Listen a lot. Listen until you understand how the image/reality, fantasy/foreplay give-and-take flows. Meantime, say little, and be completely honest in the little that you do say. This will keep you out of trouble–socially, emotionally, and sexually.

Rule Three: Realize that you are playing a role and wearing a costume. All the world, so the saying goes, is a stage, and it is no less true in a leather bar than anywhere else. The difference is that leathermen know and admit this fact, then go on to take their roles very seriously. Role-playing among leathermen is neither superficial nor changeless. When chasing sex, you and all other people play roles. You have learned to adjust your roles for maximum effectiveness, to get what you want. The difference that matters most here is that leathersex roles don't evaporate under the streetlights outside the bar. The role a man plays in the bar or other social setting (Top or bottom, cop or punk, biker or cowboy; into bondage, watersports, wrestling, or whatever) represents his considered choice of what is right for him at that time, and it is his intention that you take his image as himself at that time. In a sense, this "what you see is who I am" posture is real, the only relevant reality.

There is the heart of the matter: Leathermen are playing their roles for themselves, from something in themselves which is often of powerful importance to them, and they are looking for a proper counterpart. In nonleather circumstances the bar role is often a "play" intended for the other person, usually by someone who is much less definite about what he is looking for.

Rule Four: Don't disturb the scene! This is the paramount rule of leather bars and private leather parties. The fact that it used to be enforced rather rigorously is the source of most of the "bad press" the bars have ever had–more of the steam mentioned earlier. This rule means no loud colors, no loud voices, no perfumes, nor any of the stuff that you will instinctively understand is out of character for a leather bar. Yes, this rule is oppressive to some people, people who must squeal "Oh, Dorothy Gale, whatever kind of Kansas have you brought me to?" for instance. Even though some details of this rule are being greatly relaxed in some leather venues–particularly at daytime beer busts and such–people who fail to understand and respect the spirit of the rule do not belong in a leather bar or anywhere else in the leather scene.

Maybe if you knew just *one* of the reasons for Rule Four, you'd understand its importance. Refer to Rule Three and the comments above about negotiation becoming very sexual. There are "scenes" in progress all around you when you are among leathermen in a bar or other erotically charged setting. Men are doing the work of being who they need to be at that time. The right environment–without perfumes and loudness of clothing or behavior–makes it possible for all the scenes to coexist until the appropriate connections are made, even though many of the scenes–if broadcast–would be destructive to others going on just a few feet away.

DRESSING FOR ACTION

Black leather is an intriguing part of the leathersex and SM world. It is everywhere, and it is important, but it is not essential. There are men in the scene who never wear leather, including the heaviest and most interesting Top I ever knelt before. And there are many men in leather, some with definite sexual fetishes connected with the feel or smell of leather, who are not into rough sex at all.

If you're new to the scene, you need to consider very carefully what you are doing before you go out and spend a lot of money on leather. You can make some very expensive mistakes by dropping into a leather store and "costuming" yourself for the bar. And besides the expense, you can create some very sticky, embarrassing situations for yourself. People do this all the time, but you, not wanting to cause confusion that will get in the way of getting laid, will not be one of the men who shop first and correct their mistakes later.

Until you feel settled into a circle of leathermen, or you have spent enough time around leather-involved people to understand what your choices mean about yourself, buy only the most basic items or none. In the old days, which were not so long ago, newcomers were expected to earn their leathers. This usually involved a ritualized recognition of your "baptism" in the scene, according to the ways of the particular crowd you were moving into. For better or worse, that idea is pretty much gone, but it is still a good idea to apply to yourself. As you discover what you are into, let this rule apply: Perform now, reward yourself with the appropriate leather clothing or toy later, unless you hook up with a Daddy or Master in the meantime who wants to take charge of that for you.

Boots, levis, a belt, and a T-shirt will do, of course. It is not a problem if you don't have a jacket, vest, chaps, gloves, cap, leather pants, or sex toys to display on yourself, or hardware to signal your sexual tastes. On the other hand, it is a problem if you go out and buy yourself a leather harness, or start wearing leather neck gear (like a dog collar or knotted thong) without understanding what you are saying by your choice.

Harnesses say a lot about you, even though we are seeing a lot of them worn these days by people who obviously have no idea what they are saying. And only the "right" harness has any but a decorative use. Basically, what it comes down to is that Tops wear harnesses that are designed almost exclusively to decorate and accentuate their physiques. Very few Top's harnesses have built-in cock rings or any but the plainest straps running up the crack of the butt. Certainly, no harness made for a Top has a built-in butt plug or snaps/rings to accommodate one. A bottom's harness usually has restraining rings of some kind which can be used either to tie the bottom to himself (ring to ring) or to something else (ring to wall or dungeon furniture). Cock rings, butt plugs, front and rear chastity straps of various designs, and tough enough leather to take the abuse of being the central web of a bondage arrangement are common features of a bottom's harness. Studs are more common on the harnesses of Tops than those made for bottoms, and the heavier the studding the more likely that the harness was properly made for a Top.

Wearing almost anything around your neck is a sign, one way or another, that you are taken or owned, meaning that you will very likely not be the one to buy or install any neck gear on yourself, anyway. The act of putting a collar, especially a dog collar, on a boy used to be very important. Tops did it (apart from temporary collaring in a private scene) specifically to mark and announce their acceptance of responsibility for the collared boy. In recent years, a lot of guys have been putting collars around their own necks, going off to the bar thinking that their neck gear will assure interested Tops that they are available for fairly heavy scenes of domination and abuse. The Tops, not infrequently older and experienced in earlier ways for which they still have a great deal of respect, see the collars and steer clear. The message they get is that the boy is someone else's, at least for the night.

In recent years, on the East Coast, guys have been putting collars around their own necks, always using collars with locks on them, and leaving the locks open. The intention is to say something like, "I am available; you can be the one to close the lock." This is a hard behavior to accept because it is difficult to see whether a lock is open or closed in bar light. Besides it seems (to my antique leather sensibilities in any case) that the bottom's collar is an act of presumption. His collar or my own, which will we use? His lock–meaning *his* keys–or my own? may be a more pointed question.

Many things in leather are changing, as they always do, but some things are so useful and reasonable that it really is worth a certain amount of effort to stand against the tide of change. Harnesses are not a problem because, no matter what each player spends on wrong harnesses along the way, a good harness that reads correctly is so useful that just about everyone settles into the right style eventually. Wearing the wrong harness just isn't worth the bother of explaining yourself to everyone who speaks to you.

Collars are another matter. It is very easy for a boy who wants to say that he is available for heavy use to do so with a collar, without putting off the careful signal readers. The way to do this is to put the collar on the (right for bottom) shoulder. If you wear a leather jacket and it has epaulets, the collar can be threaded under the epaulet, under the arm, and closed. It stays in place, looks cool, and clearly says "use this" or "use me as you would a boy who wears your collar." The same treatment can be applied to whips, crops, rods, and other toys. Bring them along to demonstrate your interest, and keep them attached on your right side to demonstrate that you want them used on you. Don't overstate your interests though, and don't feel you need to bring everything with you.

For the basics of levi/leather bar and street wear–the boots, levis, belt, and T-shirt–normal and reasonable restraint will do. No flashy colors or outlandish styling are appropriate in any of it, but that certainly doesn't mean that you must look just like everyone else. Style is appreciated no less by leathermen than by anyone else, but flashiness for its own sake is generally considered more humorous than hot.

Most leather vests are perfectly safe purchases, but be sure to buy top-quality leather that can withstand sweat and sun, and shop in the shops that leathermen go to. National chains offer leather vests that are handsome enough in their way, but they stand out like Easter bonnets in a crowd of leathermen. Of course, that may be either just what you want or something you are willing to deal with for the sake of the vest or other stylish garment you really like. No problem. You will and must do what makes you comfortable, but it is wise when choosing to go against the grain to expect a few splinters.

As for the boots, unless you are ready to put up with a lot of ribbing, the only completely acceptable footgear are black boots (kept black) or black high-top shoes. In this regard, the unpardonable sins (which you may *still* choose to commit) are white shoes, especially canvas ones, and brown shoes or boots worn with black leather clothing. Extremely high heels to give yourself a lift will not go unnoticed in leather circles, and whether they are ridiculed or ignored is a matter of how well you wear them. You should understand that perfectly polished, shiny, well-kept boots will suggest, to many experienced leathermen, either a boot fetish or an interest in providing or receiving boot service of some kind. If that is not an interest, though, it doesn't mean your boots should be left shabby. Still, if you are obsessive about the look of your boots in public, don't be surprised if men expect that you are going to be obsessive about boots in the playroom.

A straightforward belt, studded or not, but not overly metallic is completely reasonable. Generally speaking, Tops who wear heavily studded belts mean to use them. Bottoms who wear heavily studded belts expect to have their own belts or similar toys used on them. Probably the most completely generic belt for a leatherman is the standard military or police issue belt with the embossed basket-weave pattern. It is a good combination of sheen and dulling pattern, has a plain steel buckle, and conveys no particular message.

Finally, the jacket: This the only expensive item you should seriously consider buying at the very outset of your career in leathersex. Leather jackets have become so fashionable that you may even already have one. If so, whatever it is, it will be fine for leather bars, social situations, etc., unless it is very trendy and *"GQ."* You know what I mean. One reason to seriously consider a jacket as an early purchase is that it will be very handy if you are asked to ride home on the buddy seat of a motorcycle. It also provides plenty of useful pockets so you don't have to ruin the contours of your ass or crotch with rings of keys, handfuls of change, or other necessities.

Just about the only way to go completely wrong in buying a leather jacket is to be overly stylish. If you go to a good store that is intent on serving the leathersex community, you will see more choices and styles than you probably guessed were possible–from "outlaw biker" to "nightclub prowler" and beyond in both directions. None of these, except possibly the ones that mix black leather into a cowboy ("brown leather") styling, are going to cause you any trouble in the bars or clubs. Ask questions. Trust the men who work in the leather stores to give correct and reasonable advice, but realize that you are ultimately responsible for your own choices. Shop with the idea of buying something comfortable that makes you look hot.

While wearing the wrong leather is not likely to cause you any trouble that can't be negotiated away in a bar or at a party, wearing no leather until you are sure of what you want is a fine, totally trouble-free option. As with everything else in the leathersex scene, when buying clothes and toys, lead with your head. Think. Examine yourself. Learn what is going on before you lay down your cash, or put your ego on the line by wearing your new leathers into a bar.

COMMUNICATING WITH CLOTHING

The clothing, portable toys, hankies, piercings, chains, boots and other things a leatherman wears are communications, as mentioned above. They tell you if he's a Top or a bottom, what his sexual tastes include, and how heavily into SM he is within his areas of sexual activity. Sometimes, especially with men under 40, the signals will seem to clash until you learn to *know* what you're looking at.

Pitfall number one: Misinterpretation. It is very easy to misunderstand the signals you get looking at men who are not well-versed in the rules of the "old leather" communities. If you have learned your leather grammar from old magazines (even some new ones) or from a friend who has been into the scene for a long time, you're idea of Tops and bottoms may be more rigid than is prevalent in bars and clubs today. These days guys switch back and forth pretty freely, almost always saying "it depends on who I am with." This sometimes results in the same guy wearing this hankie or that on the right or left depending on . . . say, what else he has in his pockets. So, misconstruing his message doesn't necessarily mean that you've forgotten your leather grammar. Instead, it means that he is ignoring his.

More misinterpretation: Except for a few hankie colors, the meaning of just about everything leathermen wear and carry can be quite different from one place to another–as with the East and West Coast versions of collar-wearing discussed earlier. This means that what you learned from *The Leatherman's Handbook* (Larry Townsend, 1972) or *Drummer* magazine may need to be reworked for your town, your club, or your crowd. For instance, in a smaller leather community (I am thinking of Las Vegas), heavily studded, hard leather and a lot of "Road Warrior" hardware can mean the man is into SM, pure and simple. The same things would mean not just SM, but very heavy, very extreme trips if they were seen at a bike club run out of San Francisco or at a bar in Chicago. The rule seems to be that in smaller or newer leather communities, where the larger percentage of guys in leather are *just* into the leather itself, sexual messages have to be bolder. So, learn from your own community.

Pitfall number two: Mistaking interests for requirements. If a man is wearing a black hankie, chances are extremely good that it will take some SM to satisfy him. Don't offer the guy a chance to neck with you unless you intend to play rough. And, if a guy is covered with leather and steel restraints, all ready to be hooked into a frame or suspension chains, he probably means it. He wants bondage of some sort, although he might accept rope bondage if that's what you're into. But almost all "special interest" signals–yellow or red hankies (for piss and fisting), handcuffs (worn right or left), a paddle hanging from the belt–should be understood as simply part of the man's sexual language, not necessarily every-night needs.

Take all these things as points to be considered and discussed. Don't mistake them for absolute requirements. Suppose a guy is wearing a red hankie in his left pocket, and you just aren't interested in being fisted, or are not "yet" ready for it. Suppose he's a hot man; in fact, excepting that red hankie, he's just the man for you. Two things suddenly become important: One, you can't just steer clear of him because it happens that he has one act in his sexual repertoire that isn't a match with your interests; and, two, talking through this point becomes essential before you get into a scene with this man. Chances are he'll accept your limits regarding fisting, but he has worn his hankie and has every right to expect that *if you don't talk to him about it* you share that interest.

Pitfall number three: Assuming that your own messages have been read and understood. Until you are known pretty widely in the circle you choose to party with, talk out your sexual intentions with men you meet as though they could know nothing from seeing your hankies, whips, or whatever. Imagining that a guy must have seen the red hankie in your right pocket could work out badly. In the darkness of the bar, it may have looked black. He may have seen it only in the glow of a yellow "bug bulb," meaning that it could have appeared orange (anything goes) or even brown (scat).

The man you are talking to may know less than you guess about any sort of sexual signaling. He might not even know that right is for bottoms, left for Tops. He might not understand that the studded strap and chain hanging from your left belt loop indicate that you expect him to *want* to wear a dog collar and leash. He may not realize that piercings, like hankies and other clothing-related signals, *can* have a left- and right-reading meaning. Maybe your man of the hour (or minute) comes from a place where a purple hankie just means you're gay (I'm thinking of small towns in Canada a long time ago, but it could still be true somewhere).

All the pitfalls of sexual signaling by our clothing and the things we carry with us to parties, bars, and clubs may make them seem useless. Not at all. You will see that the real use of the signals is not final definition, but a first communication, a starting place. With time, they will become more useful to you. If nothing else, a hankie flagging out of a hip pocket can be a reason to say, "Excuse me, Sir, in this light I can't be sure what color the hankie in your left pocket is." A beginning.

ALL DRESSED UP AND . . .

While leather bars are the most obvious places to go when you want to be among leathermen, and leather or SM clubs provide the obvious opportunities to play, there are other options. Some other possibilities will present themselves in your area. Maybe there will be a special leather-friendly weekend at a local resort, or a series of classes or lectures on sadomasochism. There could be a book signing by a major leathersex author, or a convention of manufacturers and retailers of erotic fashions. If you keep your eyes open, no matter where you live, something will come up relatively nearby, sooner or later.

Meantime, there are also some events worth going out of your way for. Some of the established annual events attract many thousands of leathermen from all over the country to a single city for three or four days at a time. You could practically plan to go where the leathermen are for every three-day weekend of the year. Presidents' Day weekend would be Pantheon of Leather (originally in Los Angeles, but now moving each year), Memorial Day weekend would be International Mister Leather in Chicago, and Columbus Day weekend would be NLA International's annual Living in Leather Conference which is staged in various cities. Also there are major leather events in many cities in conjunction with Gay Pride parades, and the international finals of the Mr. Drummer competition in San Francisco in September each year.

The Mr. Drummer finals and International Mister Leather, like many of the larger events, have become magnets attracting enough other leather celebrations around themselves that the end of May in Chicago and the third or fourth week of September in San Francisco are full-scale leather pride weeks. If nothing else, being where a lot of leathermen are–and in a party mood to boot–is a good way to find someone who wants just what you've got to give.

An even more erotically charged option is to go on a run with a bike club. (Well, usually, even though there are a few bike runs that don't exactly emphasize sex.)

CLUB RUNS

Staking out territory with the Conquistadors, frolicking in the wilds with Satyrs, and diving into the Inferno with Hellfire natives are not impossible fantasies. They are just poster-language invitations to "runs"–real events you might enjoy. Leathermen, bikers, and SM players stage runs of all sorts, getting together for a day, a weekend, or longer periods to do the things they like to do with people they like to be around.

If sex is the only thing that comes to your mind when you hear of a run, slow down and think again. Frankly, the first thing you ought to think of is a motorcycle. The earliest runs were bike club runs, often for bikers only or for "bikers and buddies," meaning that each biker could bring a buddy rider on the motorcycle with him. Some clubs still have bike runs that are only open to men on bikes. Others cling a bit to this tradition, but make certain exceptions. A run could be, for example, bikers only, but with positions for others who go ahead to prepare the meals or set up the run site.

Many clubs today, however, have given up entirely on the idea of the motorcycle as a requirement, basically just hosting a party with the special conditions that make a run a run. Even if those conditions are just about impossible to define, there is a certain feeling of camaraderie, a special sense of belonging together and having something in common, that turns a weekend camping trip for 12 to 200 men into a run.

What you will see and experience at a run depends very much on the nature of the sponsoring club. Bike clubs tend to include events that turn the whole affair into something of a motorcycle version of a rodeo. Competition in all kinds of straight and stunt riding are programmed into the run, often including some pretty strange trick riding events where buddy riders may be picked up or dropped off along the way. Cross-country scavenger hunts and riverbed races, parades with bikes dressed to the nines, and how-slow-can-you-go competitions can be expected.

When an urban leathermen's club hosts a run, the accent tends to fall more on the party than on biking, giving an atmosphere that ranges from Greek wedding to turn-of-the-century circus, often including the staging of a play, variety show, or musical evening (which is seldom taken very seriously). Drag shows are common, but it isn't often drag in the same way that you see it in vanilla bars. It's more like what your father may have done in the military service, like the show in *South Pacific*–coconut breasts and rag mop wigs on men who have no intention of looking like women. But nothing is definite, everything is possible. So, of course, serious drag can happen too.

SM clubs and organizations usually turn entirely away from the traditions of the motorcycle run, shifting the balance more in the direction of a play party. That is, for SM groups, the run is often an opportunity to do SM in a safe, supportive setting over several days and nights, often with the rare opportunity to play outdoors as a major attraction. This, in itself, actually echoes the earliest concept of the bike run pretty closely. Bikers went on runs to get to a place where they could exercise their passion for biking along with other bikers, without censure or the usual social limitations. Just so, the SM run removes from the view of the public what the public doesn't want to know about, reserving and facilitating it for those who want to experience it.

That effort to save the public the bother of protesting and being offended can sometimes mean that men who are new to the scene don't hear about all the runs that happen even in their local area. You have to meet the producers of the bike and SM runs at least halfway by looking for their posters in the right places, asking experienced leathermen at any time of year when there are significant runs, and by writing to clubs (if you can't find them any other way) to ask if they produce any events you might like to know about. Along the way, of course, you're very likely to collect more friends in leather and more information about the world of leathersex, and to put yourself in touch with functioning networks of leathermen in your hometown.

Chapter Two

Playing with Power and Sex

WHAT IS SM?

Where rough, man-to-man sex stops being butch sex and becomes SM is a question that every man answers for himself, probably differently at different times. By recognizing the power exchanged between two men in intimate circumstances, any and all of it can be called leathersex. By concentrating on other aspects–passion and arousal rather than action–some people can do just about anything they like and call none of it leathersex or SM. However you define your sexual interactions, you are probably over the line into SM sometimes in someone else's view. So, power and sex, powerful sex, and sexual power exchanges get mixed together a good deal.

The only realistic way of determining when rough sex has become leathersex is to accept each interacting pair's definition of its own action. If two men say they aren't doing SM, they're just fuck buddies, so be it, even if belts and paddles are used. If two guys call themselves a Top and a bottom, suggesting the framework of leathersex, so be it, regardless of how they have sex, and how little pain or power may be involved.

TOPS AND BOTTOMS

If leathersex is self-defined by the players, and if their acceptance of the role of Top and bottom in relation to one another is the key factor, it would be wise to know something of what the labels represent. Like most of the language around leathersex, though, the words Top and bottom, while they have definite meaning in any given circumstance, can be fairly ambiguous in general use.

A pair of generally applicable definitions–nearly useless in action, but not pointless in conversation–would go something like this: A bottom is a man whose consent to another man's action is required for a leathersex scene to happen. A Top is a man who sets before himself the goal of continually seducing another man's consent to the action in progress. Tops who are very good can seduce consent at levels that surprise and thrill the bottoms they play with. Bottoms who are very good need the most skillfully seductive Tops.

To bottom generally means to allow what someone else does. To Top means knowing what to do, how to do it, and when. So it is not surprising that new SM players almost always start as bottoms. By allowing Tops to use them, they learn technique, scene construction, safety, and the finer, less obvious facets of leathersex dynamics. Some eventually discover the desire to Top in themselves. Despite tremendous social pressure against anyone redefining himself, a new Top will emerge when a bottom's desire to take charge, his will to dominate, and his technical skill are sufficient. This is sometimes a matter of self-assertion, but it is also frequently true that men move into Topping, at least occasionally, when they are invited to do so by interested bottoms.

After a number of experiences as a Top, a man will necessarily review his performance. If it has pleased him to do what he did, and he believes he did well or could learn to do well, he may become an exclusive Top. Not all bottoms become Tops, but with very rare exceptions, Tops learn their skills and hone their scene senses by being bottoms first.

Some Tops are real man-tamers, looking to dominate unruly, self-determined bottoms who will resist their every move. Other Tops want cooperative bottoms who spell out their tastes and limits in great detail, then work with the Top to produce the scene that fulfills their wishes. Either way, the Top is the provider of stimulation, and at least nominally, the man in control once the scene begins. Tops are served by bottoms, bottoms provide service to Tops. In simple scenes this is clear and true, in more intense and more complex scenes, the truth of the matter is unchanged at some deep level, but can be warped or invisible on the surface of the visible action.

Tops, it is generally believed, are sadists, but that isn't necessarily the case. Not all leathersex involves sadistic and masochistic action. Power can be exchanged, service demanded and given, and even a certain amount of rough stimulation can be involved where no sadism or masochism is present. The Top equals sadist, bottom equals masochist equation balances as well as it needs to for each interaction. Certainly if there is to be any sadomasochistic action—giving and taking of pain for the sake of erotic pleasure–the sadist as defined by the action will be the Top as defined by the relationship. A bottom may dislike and even refuse to bear any pain, and still be a bottom, just as a Top may not enjoy inflicting pain, and may refuse to become involved in a pain scene of any sort.

A Top may be sadistic, dominant, or even very passively pleased to be served. Any combination of these factors (and others, no doubt) may properly define a given Top at a given time. Similarly, a bottom may be masochistic, submissive, or even just very eager to serve, and ready to do so from his own unaided will. A Top sometimes does all the fucking and provides the cock for all the cock sucking in a scene or a leathersex relationship, but some Tops like to suck cock and to be fucked, and may let their bottoms fuck them, or give their bottoms blow jobs sometimes, changing nothing in the definitions they have of each other as Top and bottom.

In the end, a Top or bottom does what he does, no matter what it is, and remains a Top or bottom so long as the respective bottom(s) or Top(s) he plays with see him as such. The better a man knows the leathersex scene, the more clearly he can determine what is Top action, and what is bottom action, but there are always surprises in the less-traveled outer reaches of the scene.

THE POWER EXCHANGE

This is the classic puzzle at the very heart of leathersex: the power exchange. This single, mysterious factor is vital to the safety and sanity of all acts of leathersex. It is possible for Tops and bottoms to satisfy and enjoy each other only because the power exchange works.

A simple definition of the power exchange would be a great help to everyone coming into the leather scene. Sadly, it is not possible to give a simple definition. The best we can do is to take a tour of the subject.

The power exchange is a psychological-spiritual-sexual contract between two men that defines their roles and their relationship. It can last for a few minutes or for a lifetime. Unlike any other contract though, this one is never signed. Its terms are never settled. Every gesture, every sound, every audible breath can be either a confirmation or a renegotiation of the essence of the contract. Consciously for the more experienced, less consciously for the novice, the power exchange is the context of every leathersex act, including the unspoken fantasies that have their subtle effects on the actual scene at hand.

The power exchange is the entirely voluntary process by which a bottom relies on trust, first to express his will, then to relinquish it. It is the system through which a Top accepts the responsibility represented by his bottom's surrender and promises to treat that surrender according to the ever-changing terms of the arrangement between the two of them, within the bounds of the scene. It is also the matrix of relevant facts and desires that make it possible for a bottom to express needs that develop during the scene, and expect that his communication will at least reach the Top's awareness. And it is the backdrop against which a Top, at times, can become the servant of his bottom's needs without giving up his superior position.

Both men must enter into leathersex equally dedicated to delivering themselves and each other into the greatest possible fulfillment the scene permits. Otherwise, there is no power exchange. If the Top's sadism is *only* self-serving, his acts become brutality, not sex. If the bottom's masochism is *only* self-focused, he invites either brutality or phoniness, and precludes real leathersex.

In the same way, if either man comes into the scene with only the other's needs in mind, he will prevent the power exchange from being set up, and he will undermine the safety and sanity of the scene. A Top who thinks only of the bottom's desire to be whipped, for instance, can go beyond safe and sane sensuality, in effect giving too much. A bottom desperately intent on submitting to the Top's desires without having set anything in motion for himself creates an even more unsafe situation. He is going to encourage the Top to proceed and to set aside all normal and responsible restraints and cautions.

Safety and sanity in leathersex are products of the power exchange that depends on an unconditional commitment to some agreeable form of consensuality. This is the way of leathersex: We keep the terms of the power exchange functioning–enacted fantasies of rigidity and violence notwithstanding–so that everyone gets the pleasure and experience he wants. All that said, still, we are without a definition.

Paradoxically, when the power exchange is functioning properly, the bottom is in charge of the beginning of the scene. By his desires, the contents of his relinquished will, and his limits, he defines the scope and style of the upcoming erotic action. But, once a bottom has communicated all this and confirmed his trust in the Top, control passes to the Top. This is the only predictable stage of the power exchange, and the most blatant.

Once the scene has begun, the decision-making power passes very subtly from the Top to his bottom and back. If the Top tightens up with concern or apprehension, or for any reason, he is preventing the exchange from functioning. His bottom will become tense or frightened (and rightly so). End of scene! If the bottom becomes demanding or pushy in a way that interferes with the power exchange–especially about details that were not included in the original contract, the negotiation–the Top will feel his superior position has been undermined. End of scene!

End of scene? Not necessarily physically, but the scene that was in progress, the one based on a demanding and rewarding flow of energies and wills, is gone. If the two men continue to play anyway, it is at their own risk. No mysterious power of understanding is in the wings to protect them.

In highly verbal scenes, the power exchange is easy. Without even thinking of it, Top and bottom are constantly revealing their experience of the exchange in progress. Less verbal scenes really require a more experienced Top, a less intense level of SM action, or a much slower pace to remain safe. Obviously, the way to learn about the intricacies of the power exchange is through experience, but a novice bottom ought to remember from the first that there is an exchange in progress. And he should be ready to encourage and actively (but submissively) participate in it.

This give-and-take that makes safe, sane leathersex possible always remains a bit mysterious, regardless of the experience level the players bring to the scene. One of the mysteries about the power exchange that is never completely unraveled, but must be considered, is the question of when the exchange begins. Does it start when two or more men arrive at the play space? Does it begin earlier than that, or kick in at some later moment, on demand, when the sexual or SM action reaches an otherwise unsafe intensity?

This question is *almost* in the range of things that have to be marked "unanswerable," things that you can only actually know by experience, and then only in provisional ways. It is almost, but not entirely, in that category, and the bit of it that can be discussed can also be very important to you. So, even though there is no rock-solid answer to the question, we will begin as if the correct response were: The power exchange begins with the first eye-contact between you and a potential sex partner. That is not true, your experience will prove it wrong time and again, but it is a starting point.

The reason it is important for you to accept the usually incorrect answer above as you start building your leathersex and leather scene experience is this: Until your sensitivities and understanding are developed to a certain degree, you may think that you are not yet communicating anything significant to someone else while he is sure you have already begun to *play* with him, and that you have told him a great deal about the relationship you and he are entering. By supposing that the power exchange has begun on contact, you will alert yourself to the fact that you are making meaningful gestures, saying words that can be understood as more than bar chat, and that you are (or might be) establishing the groundwork of the scene, a groundwork that will become more obvious in the following minutes or hours.

Of course, you *are* necessarily doing these things. You are supplying information about yourself and collecting information about your potential partner. This is true in any cruising or sizing-up phase. The difference is that in leathersex, you may be effectively "having sex already." That is, for instance, the Top you are communicating with may already be Topping you, and you may already be submitting to him. If you think that the power exchange starts later, you may be getting in deeper than you expect, sooner than you notice. You may be setting yourself up to look like a prick-tease, or putting yourself in a position where the negotiation of limits and acts will be compromised.

None of these problems will be all that difficult to get out of early in your leathersex experience because your tentativeness will prevent you from making really strong statements, whether you make them verbally or through nonverbal cues. The danger that does exist, apart from disappointing a Top or getting into an embarrassing situation, is that by the carelessness of your communications you may have undermined the other man's ability to trust you as completely as he needs to for the scene you might both have in mind. You might do a bit of macho strutting or submissive cowering, for example. Maybe it is inspired by a sense of discomfort that you could have washed away with the next beer. Meantime, however, to your man of the moment it may have seemed to be within the power exchange, basic to the way he adjusts himself on his side of the seesaw, and indicative of what he "should" expect of you.

Usually, if a bottom finds that the power exchange has gotten mucked up, gotten off to a bad start, it is not too difficult to fix. A bottom can always clarify his intentions, limits, willingness to submit to whatever it is, or express his newfound will *not* to submit. Any Top who will not accept the necessary restatements of the bottom's views on these things is not to be trusted. On the other hand, a bottom who tries to use what has just been said as authorization to be pushy, and unfaithful to the degree of submission he has already promised, is a cursed creature that no Top should be afflicted with.

When a Top's first moves have either been careless–which is very rare in confirmed Tops–or have been misinterpreted because the bottom did not yet realize that the scene had begun, the mess is not so easily fixed. A bottom may say "please" or "please, Sir" and get permission to speak, keeping the scene alive as it is adjusted, fixing his mistakes for his own safety. That being the case, you might think a Top could just change what needs changing and fix what needs fixing after his own initial mistakes. But, no. Because the power exchange begins basically as a current of release from the bottom and of control from the Top, extreme adjustments of the Top's role bear a special kind of danger. They are akin to *Star Trek*'s Captain Kirk appearing indecisive on the bridge. They ruin everything, most importantly trust.

We are not talking about rules or roles here, we are talking about the spiritual and psychological realities that occur naturally in a well-oiled leathersex scene. It's still confusing, isn't it? But, you were warned it would remain mysterious. All will be clarified by experience. You'll see.

PERSONALITIES AND THE POWER EXCHANGE

People who are not involved in leathersex usually assume that Tops are dominant personalities and bottoms are submissive personalities. Alternatively, it is widely believed that Tops are submissive personalities compensating in their sex lives for the weaknesses that inform the rest of their lives, and bottoms are dominant personalities performing a similar compensating ablution of their psyches. In fact, these generalizing misconceptions often get in the way of men who are attracted to the scene. A man, for instance, may feel that his sexual tastes and psychological make-up are at war if he sees himself as a bottom, but is a "my way or no way" kind of man.

Fortunately, the power exchange that makes leathersex work safely and sanely can easily accommodate both dominant bottoms and submissive Tops, and rein in both dominant Tops and submissive bottoms when necessary. There really isn't a problem here at all, nor is this necessarily only a leathersex question.

In vanilla sex, the same circumstance arises. A man may be quite demanding about being the vanilla equivalent of a bottom–"French active, Greek passive." No problem. He just sees to it that the more submissive personality he is getting into bed with understands his "demands" from the outset. The resolution is no more difficult in leathersex scenes as long as both men have been scrupulously honest at their meeting. Dishonesty, no matter what its excuses, can create insurmountable problems.

A Top with a submissive personality, for instance, can set up a sticky situation if he thinks he has to play at being the dominant personality. Besides complicating matters with his dishonesty, he will necessarily deny himself satisfying sex. By promoting himself as a dominant personality in the early stages of the power exchange, he will almost inevitably end up being matched with a submissive bottom. The result is two submissive personalities in the sex-play space together, each waiting for the other to get things rolling. Sooner or later they will either give up, or one of them will overcome his own nature and take the lead.

A bottom who covers up the truth of his dominant personality creates a similarly clumsy situation. This situation results in two dominant personalities making sexual demands on each other, with neither of them able to "give in" naturally.

Of course this sort of mismatching is not always the result of dishonesty. Around last call in a leather bar it isn't uncommon for two men to find each other attractive enough that they can agree to work out the apparent problem. The men also might be together as a result of a slave auction, a blind date, plain old desperation to get laid, or a simple mistake in the reading of signals. Or it might be that they just care enough for each other to put in the extra effort that may be required.

Regardless of how the situation arises, there are at least three ways that two dominant or two submissive personalities can put the power exchange on track and have super leathersex anyway. First, they can just talk it out. Since this can mean quite a lot of talking, it's a good idea to make the talk "hot," meaning the scene gets a strong verbal start.

Another relatively easy method can be borrowed from the usual habits of some men who, under certain conditions, switch between being Tops and bottoms: Ritualize the beginning of the power exchange as a "struggle" (a wrestling match, for example) that will determine the general course of the sex scene to follow. The winner of the struggle, it is agreed, will outline the scene he wants. Of course, if the bottom wins (how clumsy, but it could happen), he has to be true to his desires and cast himself in the role of the bottom in the scene he creates. This sounds a bit sticky, but it isn't. If, for example, the scene is to be a fantasy, a bottom could cast himself as any one of many historic figures who were absolutely in charge of their own flogging or other punishments (monks of The Inquisition, Henry II after the death of Becket, etc.).

Yet another simple resolution of the clash between two dominant or two passive personalities trying to get it on is to agree, without staging a struggle, to have the leathersex scene within a fantasy that straightens out the roles and establishes the first few moves in the game. In this situation, whether the man cast in the Top role is a dominant or submissive personality, he *has* to play his part. A submissive Top is then serving his submissive nature by taking the lead in the scene, submitting to its demands, without putting an inappropriate control in the hands of the bottom. Similarly, a dominant bottom's nature can be answered by the right fantasy role, making it possible for him to be "overcome" by the Top even if the Top is a submissive personality.

So, when a situation develops that puts two personalities of the same "stripe" into a sexual pairing with each other, they can talk it out, "fight" it out, or act it out with a fantasy scene. Then, once a workable set of first-stage ground rules is in effect, the power exchange, with little more than the usual attention, will take its course, leading to (or at least tending toward) a mutually satisfying experience for all concerned.

In the final analysis, the power exchange teaches most of us to balance dominant and submissive traits in our own personalities. So a long-experienced leatherman, Top or bottom, finds that he can be a good personality match for anyone whose bottom/Top orientation and erotic wish list of the moment is interesting to him.

LEATHERSEX AS SEX

Sometimes there is no genital sex associated with a leathersex scene, but that is relatively rare when men play at home. At public play parties and sex clubs it is not only usual but desirable that most SM encounters include SM action but little or no genital sex. After all, you might like to play with any number of Tops in the course of an evening-long play party, but do you really want to come every time? (Yes is an acceptable answer, obviously.)

At home, where two or a few men are playing together, and there is no passing crowd of other potential play partners, sex that results in orgasms is usually worked into the play at some point. On the other hand, a wildly successful leathersex scene can sometimes so far surpass the sensations of genital sex that an orgasm would be an impossible step *down* in experience. Nonetheless, cocks and their favored receptacles have a place in the leathersex scene.

In fact, a cock can have a central place in some scenes, whether it is used for insertive sex or not, or whether it is used to achieve an orgasm or not. There is cock worship, a scene that turns on a lot of Tops, and satisfies a lot of bottoms. Actually, a lot of devoted cocksuckers are silently practicing cock worship in sexual situations where they don't recognize or admit the leathersex component. They enjoy begging for and being denied the cock. They want to be ordered to touch, look at, or "taste" the cock in just this way or that. Because this sort of encounter sets up, maintains, and relies upon a full-scale power exchange, it can be understood as leathersex (which is no reason for *demanding* that guys who do this identify themselves as leathermen).

Sex involving the genitals can be a prelude to SM, giving both parties an intensely close look at each other, and a very effective opportunity to express themselves to each other. Genital sex before a heavy leathersex scene is even essential for some men who, once they come, can't handle anything sexual happening for a long time. These guys, Top or bottom, are well advised to either jerk off before the scene or see that they are "forced" to come (even "milked") before the first stages of the leather scene. Those first steps of leathersex, being both relatively less intense and significantly full of promise, are likely to be bearable, one way or another, after coming. On the other hand, the risk of coming accidentally during a scene—and not being able to continue—is lessened if the person with the don't-touch-me-I've-come attitude comes before it all gets under way.

Other people—likely the majority—see SM scenes as foreplay to be closely followed by genital sex. These guys, of course, might not like to say it quite that plainly, and might even fail to see it that way (even if things just keep working out that way). Besides, the men who do leathersex first with genital sex to follow are probably all the more satisfied if the SM portion of the evening so completely drains and exhilarates them that they "forget" to fuck and suck later.

Still others—the other potential majority—get their genital sex somewhere in the midst of the leathersex scene. If the scene is mainly about bondage, say, the bound man may be forced to suck the Top's cock or to show the Top how well he follows orders by jerking off on command, and not coming until he is given permission. The possible scenarios for fitting orgasms into leather scenes are infinite. They are, in fact, the stuff of which the fantasies of future leathermen are made.

MORE ABOUT COCKS

Of all the body parts and accoutrements of gay sex, surely the single most talked-about is the cock. And, of all the things that might be of interest about a cock, nothing seems to get as much attention as the size of the thing itself. Scientific studies have documented penis measurements repeatedly, always coming up with largely the same results: Cocks don't vary in size as greatly as people imagine (or claim), with some wildly unusual exceptions. Race is a factor, but not a reliable or extreme factor in cock size. And, supporting the rallying cry of men who think they are underendowed, size is not a major element in sexual satisfaction for the Top or bottom party in intercourse.

Before getting off the subject of size and back to the leathersex uses of cocks, one last thing must be said: For oral sex, size can be very important to the experience of both parties, but there are suckers out there looking for cocks of every possible length, thickness, shape, and color. Thank goodness.

The cock can have a very special place in leather scenes regardless of its size and other physical characteristics. While many ways of playing with cocks will be discussed in later chapters, both explicitly and by inference, it might be soothing for cock-loving leather novices to know some of the leathersex options for cock use right away. Remember, though, that SM scenes don't always include anything overtly sexual, and that a scene can also become very sexual without involving either man's cock, or involving only one of them.

Cock torture is the first thing most people come to when they combine the idea of SM with the thought of a penis. Fine, this is a good starting point. Cocks and balls can be tortured to wonderful effects by stretching, clamping, abrasion, bondage, piercing, cutting, beating, kicking, prolonged and/or controlled masturbation–in any way that just about any other body part can be tortured.

Cock torture does involve some dangers. (Catheters and sounds–tubes and rods inserted into the urethra–should not be used as pain or torture devices. Learn to use them properly before using them at all.) Generally though you can learn what you need to know about causing pain to the penis by plain old-fashioned doing. Do unto yourself what you would either do unto others or have them do unto you. That's a good safety rule. Stop when the pain is too much. Stop if the pain begins to travel into other body parts. And, by all means, take the advice and ministrations of experienced men whenever and wherever you can.

Cock sucking can be, within certain fantasy or strict role-playing contexts, a form of leathersex. Verbal scenes can be built around cock sucking and oral sex can be performed "against the will" of either party, with or without either pain or bondage to "enforce" the performance.

Still, the most purely leathersexual roles of the male organ in the playroom involve the Top's cock as goal and reward for the bottom, and/or exposing or ignoring the bottom's cock as a way of under-scoring his place in the scene. Commonly, but far from universally, the dungeon clothes of Tops include jocks or other coverings for their own genitals. Just as commonly Tops and bottoms agree that the bottom should be either naked or at least exposed, front and rear, early in the scene.

This situation–naked bottom, covered Top–puts the Top at a psychological and physical advantage that works to everyone's benefit in many ways, not the least of which is the support it gives to the power exchange. The Top has access to the bottom's body for whatever use and abuse he wants, within the limits and negotiated intent of the scene. Meantime, the bottom is able to imagine, wish for, ask for, and even beg for a chance to see, smell, touch, taste . . . eventually, perhaps, "take" the Top's cock one way or another. While all of this can be very superficial, to the extent that it reflects and expresses the power exchange in process, it becomes a way of knowing all along how the head trip and the physical scene are working.

The idea of reward and punishment as driving forces for an SM scene is not necessary at all. It is even distasteful to many leathermen. All the same, if the reward is the Top's cock, and the punishment is that the said cock is kept under wraps, nothing untoward comes of it. The most likely effect, in fact, is that the scene, no matter what actions it includes, remains charged with a very desirable sexual energy.

Obviously, cocks get used in many other ways in the play room. Faces are slapped with them, breathing is controlled by measured plunging and withdrawal, guys get fucked while they are in bondage or while they are being stimulated with pain or "humiliation," and the list goes on. All of which is pretty easily accessible to the kinky, sex-positive imagination. Perhaps the most important thing for a leathersex novice to realize is that so many different things are possible that all limiting assumptions are bad bets. The perfect rule of thumb about the penis in the playroom: Negotiate the place of your cock and his in the scene, or accept the surprises you get.

WATERSPORTS

Cocks come into leathersex power play another way, as the providers of piss. Unattractive as some people find it, piss is hot stuff to a lot of guys. Even so, piss play or watersports is one of those things, even one of those words, that embarrasses people. Why? What is so embarrassing about wanting to see, play in, drink, or be "humiliated" with piss in a subculture that accepts all kinds of variations on oral sex, rimming, and bootlicking so much more easily?

Oppressive potty training? Maybe. But, whatever causes the discomfort around watersports as a topic of conversation seems to evaporate like piss on hot concrete the moment the curtains are drawn and the lights are down. Despite the almost complete absence of yellow hankies (the flag for watersports) hanging out of hip pockets, the fact is that just about every boy you'll ever be with will either be actively seeking piss or readily willing to take it, one way or another.

The saddest thing about watersports is the lingering taboo against piss. Because of that, a lot of guys end up playing only with their own, by themselves, in the secrecy of their own homes. They never "get it," and they never share the fun with anyone.

Some people will tell you that the reason they don't "go for the gold," even though they know they want to, is that it isn't safe–especially now–in terms of infectious diseases. It may be impossible to argue that point with guys who have already made their decision, but they're wrong. Anyone who is claiming the medical "ickiness" of piss as an excuse for denying himself the pleasure of watersports is just not familiar with the facts, old or new. This is not to say that *nothing* medically undesirable can come from piss play or piss drinking. A man with a lot of alcohol or drugs in his system can intoxicate his urinal-boy. A man with a bladder or urethral infection is necessarily introducing infectious organisms to whatever surfaces he pisses on, but he's likely to be aware of the infections and lose interest in piss as play when it is uncomfortable anyway. And, there are other disease organisms that can apparently survive in human urine, which doesn't seem to stop the piss fans from playing wet games.

When the discussion of body fluids–piss specifically–turns to HIV, there is actually clear evidence that golden showers (piss on the outside of the body) and recycled water (piss drinking) are HIV safe. Studies of possible HIV transmission conducted at Tufts University and the Harvard School of Medicine as reported in *The Journal of Infectious Diseases* in December, 1989, determined that no "replication quality" HIV survived in the urine.

Ours, to bend a phrase, is not to reason why or why not, but to work on the how of pleasure. As for why you do or don't do anything, you're on your own, but here is a glimpse of what leathermen sometimes do with piss. After all, what other people call waste water is only considered a waste by some of us if it is discarded before it is shared.

Piss can be a reward: "You can't have *my* piss till you prove you deserve it." It can be a punishment: "You've been such a poor cocksucker, I'll just use you as a urinal instead." It can be a challenge given to establish or test relative degrees of dominance and submission: "Yes, here and now, in the bar, in front of your pals, piss in your faded jeans and let the piss collect in your boots." It can be, one step further in the same direction, intentional humiliation: "Now that we are sure your friends are watching, get down and beg me to piss on you. If you beg really well, I may even piss on your face." This could be followed perhaps by piss, or by the announcement that you aren't even a good place to piss. Once the submission is agreed upon and clear, it can simply be a reminding and constant duty: "When you need to piss, ask. I may give you permission to go to the bathroom, require you to piss in your pants, or order you to hold it until further notice. When I have to piss, I will tell you what to do. You may be allowed to drink it straight from the source, or catch it in a glass and either drink it or carry it to the bathroom for me, or you may be required to stretch out in the tub or on the floor and give me something to piss on."

Urination, adequately eroticized in advance, can be like coming. No, not like coming. It can be coming, the feeling of an orgasm going on and on, controllable and extendable in a way that no other orgasm can be. It can be filth or a cleansing flood. And, in the right context, piss scenes can make the liquid flow go either way, Top to bottom, bottom to Top, but the context of the latter can be tricky to maintain within the leathersex power exchange.

Surely the most powerful watersports scenes are ones in which the Top takes control of the bottom's right to piss, then "forces" in the fluid (perhaps his own piss or the bottom's) until the need becomes urgent. This gives a tremendous underpinning to any and all surrounding leathersexual activity. It raises to the level of urgency the simplest spanking or command. To stand rigid against the wall on orders can become plain old boring, but to stand rigid against the wall and resist the urge to relieve a bursting bladder is not boring at all.

Also among the ranking watersports games is the scene in which the bottom (finally!) gets his lips around the Top's cock only to discover (surprise!) that the Top pisses without warning. There is no time to rethink anything. There is no way for the bottom to ease up without blowing it. A commitment to the moment is required, immediately. And, a well-balanced Top will sometimes use this moment perfectly, despite the surprise: "Spill a drop and you'll regret it!"

If you think you're up for wet and wild as a way of having a good time, try it. Understand that you are not alone. More people are getting down and getting wet than you'll ever know from cruising hankies or asking questions. And, make your own choices about piss as you must about everything in your erotic repertoire.

One note of special significance to people who intend to provide recycled "drinking water" is in order here: You are in charge of what the bottom smells and tastes in your piss. Some drugs can still be in the piss and be active, but they don't usually change the flavor or smell. What you eat, on the other hand, has a tremendous effect on the flavor of your piss. One famous piss player in the glory days of the Caldron (the definitive San Francisco piss palace), claimed that strawberries eaten a couple of hours before a piss scene provided an irresistible, sweet piss flavor, and a lot of people with good reason to know agreed with him. Even the rascally statesman Ben Franklin had a few words to say on the subject in a satirical letter to a scientific academy: "Certain it is also that we have the Power of changing by slight Means the Smell of another Discharge, that of our water. A few Stems of Asparagus eaten, shall give our Urine a disagreeable Odour; and a Pill of Turpentine no bigger than a Pea, shall bestow on it the pleasing Smell of Violets." As for the turpentine, few modern leathermen can confirm or deny its effect, but the power of asparagus and other dark green vegetables to spoil a piss scene is famous.

NONGENITAL SEX

It is perfectly normal (if you will pardon the word) to think of sex as an activity involving the genitals and resulting in the emission of sticky white stuff. If you are male, that's the whole thing according to big brothers, Dad, your coach, or whoever it was who gave you the birds-and-bees speech, assuming someone did. But, sex is not a matter of which body part you engage, but of which energy you use.

When a doctor examines your "private parts" it might or might not be exciting. The difference may be how good looking the doctor is to you. It may be how he handles your "merchandise," and that may be a matter of how good looking you are to him. Or it may be something else. But, the very fact that Dr. A under circumstances B can fiddle with your dick without getting you sexually aroused, while a different combination of doctor and circumstances can leave you with a raging, aching hard-on is a hint that there is something beyond contact with a particular body part involved in the whole procedure.

Some guys can come from being fucked, others have to help themselves along. Some bottoms will sometimes come from being whipped, others find that whipping is only foreplay that must be followed by some sort of genital action. Still, somewhere in the mix of action and imagination that makes up sexual arousal and raises it to a climax, every one of us can identify the details in our own experience that prove that sex is not necessarily a genitals-only experience.

In leathersex, especially when groups of men play together, it is (oddly?) often the Top whose genitals never get into the action. For now, we will leave the Top to fend for himself. But, if you are a bottom, you may actually have to intentionally eroticize some nongentital contacts just to get over the programming that ignorantly defines sex as a dicks-required area of activity. To do so will be very wise for a bottom whose tastes run to whipping, bondage, verbal abuse, and other things that are already nongenital.

In point of fact, Mr. Perfect is defined by his ability to provide the very thing about which you fantasize. What bottom in his right mind involves his fantastic Mr. Perfect in the satisfaction of his own (the bottom's) cock? None, it doesn't make sense! So, you imagine your Mr. Perfect whipping you. You imagine him flooding your face or torso with warm beer. You imagine him ramming dildoes into you, or his fist, or doing whatever else confirms your position as his bottom and his position over you.

Now, while he's not around, sneak a chance to eroticize the thing you want. The more completely you do so, the more completely you will be able to convince him that you want it, are satisfied with it when you get it, and–very importantly–that, if he will just give you this, you will respect, admire, and appreciate him, and–most importantly–you will wish to see him again.

To eroticize a fist, a dildo, piss, being ignored, immobility, rope, chain, leather, or whatever, engage your example or fantasy of it at your climax when you masturbate. It really is that simple. But first, a two-fold warning: (1) don't do this if you find that the nongenital "thing" is already highly sexual to you or if you can already experience sexual satisfaction without genital involvement when this thing is part of the scene, and (2) don't do this so consistently that you make yourself totally dependent on the newly eroticized thing, and unable to come without it.

In the former case, you are wasting your time on an unneeded activity. In the latter case, you are closing doors that you may want to go through again one day. In either case, when you eroticize the object unduly, you are creating a limiting fetish, one that you will sometimes want to escape but may find yourself unable to become aroused without. You don't want to be in a state where one particular fetish is so attached to all phases of your sexual expression that you cannot experience pleasure without it. If nothing else, this bores a continuing partner.

After all, the point of understanding that sexual expression and sexual satisfaction need not be entirely genital is that you will sometimes encounter a man who wants to Top in a way that does not involve taking any interest in your cock and balls, or allowing you to do so. This, in itself, can be eroticized. But, besides being able to get turned on without demanding an orgasm, you want to be able to satisfy and to be satisfied by a man who fulfills your leather-sex fantasies, whatever they are and whatever they become. So, you have to give those fantasies access to your finest, fullest, and most potent sexual energy.

Do it. Be glad you can do it. Just be careful not to limit your sexual repertoire in the process.

FISTING

There is little doubt that fisting is sex, and there is no room to doubt that guys who are into fisting are aware of the power they are exchanging. So, by applying all the interlocking definitions, fisting is leathersex; it is playing with power.

Fisting takes a pleasure that just about every gay man understands and carries it to a level of intensity that is almost incomprehensible even for guys who do it often. In the way that the second-wind, hit-the-wall, runners' high is a complete mystery to casual joggers, fisting is beyond the ken of guys who just get fucked with dicks and dildos.

What happens when you push your hand and arm inside another man's body or when your body allows another man's hand and arm to be pushed inside, is not just fucking with a giant, organic dildo. It is a connection between two people that eases both of them through passageways of trust and caring not even suggested by ordinary genital sex. The slightest error in judging the state of relaxation, for instance, can lead to the collapse of the experience, or worse, to serious injury. So, profoundly felt trust is essential. The briefest distraction from the act at hand (pun intended, of course) can result in the bottom losing his momentum in the climb from level to level of bearable intensity. In order not to have to back off or slow down–losing hard-won sensory advantages–both men have to be sensitive to each other and the process at a very deep level.

Fisting is leathersex at its most sexual and it is one of the acts that most graphically displays the leathersex power exchange in all its details. The Top must seduce both the bottom's mind and his muscles, and constantly reconfirm that seduction, even if what he is doing is something the bottom desperately wants him to do. The bottom must constantly reassert his willingness to proceed both to the Top and to his own body.

Because of the delicate balance of consent and seduction in fisting, and because the sensations and emotions involved are so intense, fisting is one leathersex act that is almost never undertaken in a context of fantasy. Unlike whipping, for example, where the idea that the bottom is being forced, punished, or violated may heighten the experience, fisting is usually surrounded with only realistic statements and comments about getting the fist in, learning to handle it, getting what you want, and so forth. A good fisting Top will discover to what extent the bottom needs to be given the impression that he *must* accept and bear the pain associated with fisting, but he will never push the fisting to the point that any other goal surpasses the striving for mutual pleasure (with the accent on the bottom's sensations).

It is not unusual for two men to spend weeks or even months "building up" to the bottom being able to take the Top's fist–and the successes and setbacks along the way can be a pleasurable kind of erotic play. Nor is it all that unusual for a bottom to nurse the desire to be fisted for years before "risking" a serious effort, only to discover that it is actually fairly easy for him to do it with the right man at the right time and place. And, frankly, all of it–the deferred desire, the long build-up, the sudden achievement–is perfectly reflective of the power exchange and the underlying realities of leathersex.

With all the longing that often precedes it and the nearly unparalleled intensity of pain and painless sensations that accompany it, it is no wonder that fisting is the route through which many men connect their sexuality and their spirituality. Fisting is a mind-altering experience. It is an opportunity to face and conquer any lingering traces of puritanical bias against sex and pleasure. And, it is a real test of a man's ability to connect on every level with another man, in a trusting intimacy that is not usually possible with vanilla sex or necessary for most other forms of radical sex.

Fisting is also one of the leathersex possibilities that requires preparation, training, and carefully developed experience. The mental preparation is fairly obvious, and most guys who are ever going to be fisted spend lots of time silently or talkatively doing this prep work, building up a clear desire if nothing else. The physical preparation–cleaning out the bowels and providing oneself with enough grease and time and towels–is another matter, and also very important. The twin questions of training and experience can often be handled together. That is, an experienced man leads an inexperienced one, helping him deal with whatever comes up–physically, emotionally, and mentally. And the experienced man may be either the Top or the bottom. Commonly, in fact, an experienced fister takes the bottom role in training a newcomer. Then they switch after the new man has seen close-up what is possible.

Presumably, two inexperienced men can work up to and enjoy fisting, but it cannot be advised. Having been there before, especially as both a Top and a bottom, is the only way to know with a reliable degree of certainty what is predictable and acceptable pain, and what is resistance of a dangerous sort; what is the natural difficulty, and what is a clear signal that something is going wrong. Find a man who knows, and cooperate. The pleasure you're working toward is worth it, and the joy of later sharing that pleasure with other men is indescribable.

ASS PLAY

Fists aside or not, there is probably nothing about gay sex that so mystifies or repels straight heterosexuals as the fact that many of us put stuff into our own and each other's asses. Fingers and cocks and hands, dildos and vibrators and ice cubes, hoses and night sticks and coke bottles. Guys put all sorts of things "in the out" so to speak, and enjoy it. And ass play of all sorts–not just fisting–is found in the leatherman's repertoire, connecting with just about every aspect of leathersex.

To the extent that leathersex is domination-submission power play, working over an ass is a way of expressing and acting on the roles. The Top, it is generally conceded, has the right, at his discretion, to the bottom's body, even to the inside of it and even through the asshole. That, of course, is the rhetoric underlying the reality of mutual satisfaction, at least as a goal.

To the extent that leathersex is about pain, ass play is one of the options for providing a bottom with painful stimulation. This, though, gets into a slightly touchy area. When ass play is actually painful–not just a bit of a stretch, but a major pain in the ass–there is often something wrong. If the bottom's pain is not thoroughly mixed with and overcome by his pleasure, the object being inserted is too large, the wrong shape, moving too fast, insufficiently greased, or is being angled badly.

To the extent that leathersex is overtly sexual, the ass is an organ of sexual pleasure for a leatherman, just as it can be for anyone. After all, even straight men know (despite their denials) that the nerves in the area immediately around the anus are part of the same super-sensitive neural network that serves the cock and balls. But nerve-response type sensations are barely the beginning of the fun men–especially leathermen–have sticking things into butts.

At best, leathermen go about ass play with the power exchange in full working order, the sexual responses firing normally, and a good balance of pain-pleasure sensations in mind. When we do, we can really soar, but no one needs to explain how it happens to be true that doing a lot of what feels good is a great thing. What is needed is (go ahead, groan) a certain amount of caution.

Warnings are especially important when we're talking about

penetrating ass play for a number of reasons. First, the tissues inside the bowel are fairly easily cut and torn. Second, injuries to the lining of the intestine are not always immediately obvious. Third, ordinary household remedies are seldom adequate attention for the internal injuries that can occur during careless ass play.

So, at the risk of sounding like Dad shouting "keep that crayon out of your mouth," here are the basic cautions:

Don't put (or allow anyone to put) anything into your ass that is not made to go there, except when extreme caution has been exercised in choosing or modifying an object so that it is smoothed into a shape that at least roughly approximates the contours of a cock. "Roughly" can mean as cock-like in shape as, say, a fist and arm are.

Don't put up with any sharp pain that *seems* to come from inside your body when something is being inserted. Such pains can be from gas or solid matter being pushed around, which is not a safe game plan, or they can signal the threat of serious injury. On the other hand, a good deal of pain at the anal opening may be entirely acceptable. That is a matter of taste.

Finally, don't allow the speed or angle of the object being inserted or thrust in and out of your ass to remain recurrently painful. This could be the same gas or solid matter problem, but what we are actually talking about here is different. The speed-to-grease ratio, which is also very dependent on relaxation, can easily determine the likelihood of abrasion injury or slight tears in the tissue. The angle of insertion, if wrong, can also cause abrasion injuries, internal bruising, and other tears in the tissue.

Almost enough warnings, but there is one other thing you will want to consider: disease transmission. There is definitely some risk of carrying a disease from one body to another on an ass toy. There is no doubt that some disease organisms can live–whether for minutes or forever–on the surfaces of the toys or in the grease and body fluids left there. So, a reasonable precaution is to avoid these risks altogether by using condoms on your ass toys whenever possible and cleaning them thoroughly after every use. Taking the added precaution of using any given ass toy only with the same bottom is not a bad idea, if not always practical. A reasonable balance of single-ass use, careful cleaning, and condoms is something you can work out for yourself. Don't leave it to chance. Work it out consciously.

More than enough, don't you think, of warnings and don'ts. As for the other side of the coin: Do play with your ass. Do let other guys play with your ass. Do put into your ass any safely shaped object of any size you can accommodate and enjoy. Do overcome any feeling you may have that ass play is too dangerous to be enjoyed. Do share your ass with your leathersex partners, rather than thinking of it as a sex organ for vanilla encounters only. And, perhaps most important, realize that your asshole is a pretty independent area of muscles which may take a good deal of seducing. So, play with men who are willing to be patient in the process of sphincter seduction.

GROUPS, GANGS, AND MOBS

Group sex, ranging from three-ways to massive, anonymous orgies, is part of being gay for some of us. One-on-one relationships that make no concessions to this drive are doomed if one or both men involved have some kind of group-sex need, acknowledged or not. Leather sexuality, it seems, is more likely than other categories of homosexuality to include the urge to play with multiple partners either simultaneously or in bathhouse-style rapid succession, as well as embracing the freedom to have any number of partners over any period of time, even when a continuing relationship is successfully in place.

It also happens that leathersex, by its very nature, complicates the cautions and "etiquette" required for successful group sex play.

A lot of leathersex bottoms have fantasies of being used and abused by "all your friends, too," or some otherwise-defined group. It's not unusual at play parties for a Top to install his bottom as a urinal for all to use, a whipping boy to be flogged by anyone, or something of the sort. But, for all the trouble that is taken to make these situations feel out-of-control for the bottom involved, they are controlled circumstances, fantasies being fulfilled, and not the free-for-all they seem. The Top does not give up his responsibility for the bottom's safety in these situations. The bottom, on the other hand, who puts himself in a similar position, may be setting up an uncontrollable series of events.

If everyone present is actually known to be safe–an established SM club with dungeon masters on duty, for instance, or a party where all guests are from within the network of known leathermen with some provision for guests to be brought as well–there can be sufficient anonymity to realize the fantasy of a bottom being used by any number of strangers, without any great risk. The situation can be put into high gear by blindfolding the bottom to increase the anonymity and the surprise factors, of course. In a public place like a bathhouse, however, there can be some surprising dangers.

While it is understood from the beginning that group sex is a matter of personal choice, it must also be understood that gangs and mobs are not *sexual* groups at all. A gang is a group of people set against one or more other people. The result of what passes for sexual expression for a gang is brutality, not sexuality. A mob is a group of people who have lost their individual personalities, their reason, their powers of will, and their separate understandings of responsibility in the frenzy of the group's activity. Mobs may or may not do dangerous things, but there is nothing to prevent it, no presence of responsible individuality. Groups of actual strangers become gangs and mobs very easily since the bottom's anonymity reduces everyone's sense of responsibility for his safety.

Groups, perhaps excited by leathersex opportunities with which they are not familiar, can devolve into mobs. Men who start out willing to be used by a group can find themselves unexpectedly at the mercy of a gang of inept idiots.

Sometimes, at least after they get going on their dangerous tracks, the actions of a gang or mob can seem to be related to leathersex. Not so. That impression results from a novice's lack of genuine leathersex experience. You don't want to have anything to do with these abuses of sexuality that place violence (the gang) or irresponsibility (the mob) ahead of genuine mutual satisfaction (that's sex!).

If the fantasy factory in the back of your head or in the depths of your groin is telling you either gangs or mobs "sound okay to me," think again. A gang-bang fantasy can certainly be played out–and sometimes with tremendous, unforgettable pleasure all around–but it has to be within the leathersex power exchange: safe, sane, consensual sex; satisfying in context, content, and execution to all parties. A mob scene, on the other hand, is never safe and cannot safely be incorporated into a fantasy that is to be played out, if only because it necessarily involves individuals disowning personal responsibility for their acts.

A good deal of leathersex actually happens in group settings. Each setting, each club, each group has its own style, and the style is often defined in a formal set of rules that you are expected to know before you enter the play area. The best clubs actually ask that you sign a "release" that, among other things, assures the party organizers that you are aware of and agreeable to the rules of the space. Because leathersex groups often break into pairs and small groups, the most important rules often have to do with not talking about anything nonsexual in the play area, and how to leave or join a group that is already at play.

For the person who arrives alone at a leathersex play party, the rules of the space and ordinary manners are usually all that you need in order to have a safe and enjoyable experience. If you arrive with a "date," whether it is your Master, slave, lover, current leathersex fling, or "just a date," different arrangements may be required. First, if you're the bottom, the rules that govern your behavior will necessarily be all the rules of the space plus the rules of your Top. This must be discussed in advance unless you are absolutely, positively, certainly certain that the requirements are all fully understood from the context of your existing relationship. Assume nothing. To assume, as the saying goes, makes an "ass" of "u" and "me."

Secondly, if you arrive as a member of a couple, you must find a way to communicate the special circumstances of your being together to the rest of the group that will be in the play area. Many parties start with social periods, largely made up of introductions, during which the lighter mood allows these things to be explained, and this prevents a great many misunderstandings later on. During such a social period, a bottom eagerly serving a Top will be noticed and the relationship implied by service as simple as staying at his feet, running to get his coffee, etc., will explain everything.

Group sex circumstances that do not allow for the safety provided by introductions, or groups that are already in session when you and your partner join them are often a little more difficult.

In these situations you may either have to play very visibly with one another to visually communicate what you have not been allowed to say, or you may have to explain your situation to each player or group of players who become interested in you or your partner. Do it. If you don't, you risk upsetting the party for everyone, even turning a happy group into an unsympathetic gang.

POWER GAMES FOR TWO PLAYERS

Even though group scenes are interesting to a lot of people, and there are people who do SM alone, it is still true that most leathersex is one-on-one. That is, one Top and one bottom, doing together whatever they mutually agree will give them both the experience they want. Some pairs of leathermen become couples and a later chapter is devoted to their various kinds of relationships. But for most novices, it is not a particularly good idea to jump into a relationship that limits experimentation. Leathersex offers a sea of possibilities, and–unless everlasting love catches up with you–you will want to know about a lot of it before you put yourself in a situation that prevents you from finding out more about your options.

SHORT-TERM RELATIONSHIPS

Any continuing relationship that can develop between two leathermen can also be played out as a scene for a few hours, a weekend, or any limited period. Once a Top is in charge, a bottom has submitted to his will, and the basic limits have been established (including the time limits, if any) anything can happen. The Top may be the Master to the bottom as slave. If the relationship is set up to last only till midnight because one or the other has to be up for work the next day, so be it. Nothing that is real is any less real for existing in a limited time period. The bottom may become the Top's dog or horse; his footstool or doormat; his urinal or ashtray. But most usually, the bottom is just the bottom, and the Top the Top. The two of them undertake the enjoyment of erotic stimulation, at the Top's discretion and within the bottom's limits, leading to mutual satisfaction. For the most part, they play with pain or some other leathersex elements that could be just as effective in group or solo play.

Major variations on the theme of a Top and a bottom satisfying one another include switches, mutual players, and the turning of the tables.

A switch is a person who may play as Top or bottom. He often has a preference for one or the other, switching only under certain circumstances. A guy may like to be flogged, for example, but demand that he be flogged only by the best and most experienced Tops (a reasonable demand when it comes from a bottom of extensive experience). If flogging is this guy's only comfortable bottom scene, he may Top at all other times. So, it will sometimes happen that he starts the evening off as a Top, then somehow discovers that the bottom is actually expert at the other end of the whip. A little renegotiating may be required, but trust the flogging pig to be able to get what he wants when it's available, even if the purveyor is grovelling at his feet.

Mutuality is less common, but for the guys who want it, it is usually absolutely required–at least if they are going to do any Topping. In a mutual scene the rule of thumb is do unto others what they have just done or are about to do unto you. This can have all kinds of exciting possibilities. Whip fights can hardly happen between a Top and a bottom, and switches are unlikely to consider them because they want the power exchange flowing in its usual circuit during a scene, but mutual players love it. Stroke for stroke, if you can get your strokes in, both players give and take a whipping. Nipple play, watersports, spanking, ass play, fisting, and variations on oral and anal sex are all easily susceptible to mutual play. Humiliation, games of slavery, and bondage are not.

Turning the tables on a Top, scenes founded on the expectation that the bottom will be pushed to the point that he breaks free of the Top's control and reverses the action, are relatively rare. Sometimes a bottom who is forced to Top by circumstances beyond his control (usually his own discomfort with bottoming), will try to orchestrate a scene to go this way. The inherent dishonesty is distasteful to most leathermen, but it is sometimes possible (and sometimes advisable) to clue the nominal Top in so that he is expecting and accepting of the turn the scene is going to take.

Another, far less common variation on the usual Top and bottom arrangement comes up when a Top asks to be Topped. Just as most people basically didn't believe in bisexuals a few years ago–thinking they were queers who hadn't come out or straights having a fling–they now doubt that a Top who wants to be Topped from time to time is still a Top. This is a nonissue. What does complicate it, more often than not, is the submitting Top's wish for the procedure to remain a secret between himself and the selected Topper of the Top. This is an embarrassment to the whole leathersex scene. If there were not an underlying feeling that to Top is a higher and better calling than to bottom, we would not have good Tops keeping their occasional bottom needs secret. Worse yet, we would not have experienced Tops souring for lack of a feeling that they are free to have those needs met. The situation is changing in the right direction in the 1990s, but it has a lot of changing to do.

BONDAGE IN GENERAL

Among play options for two, few activities are as often undertaken as bondage. Probably the most usual sort of bondage is restraint to facilitate some other scene, but that doesn't reduce the value of the bondage as bondage. Visually and physically, it symbolizes and expresses the Top-bottom relationship. For some scenes, like flogging of the cock and balls, bondage is almost essential. For other scenes, like electro-torture, it is nearly irrelevant. For almost any scene, it turns up the leathersex thermostat very comfortably.

Apart from the useful nature of bondage as a way to restrain a bottom so he will remain exactly in place and available for some other kind of attention, there are uncounted other reasons for doing bondage in which the bondage is either the scene itself or a distinct component in its own right.

The power exchange that makes a bondage-only scene work for the Top is hard to understand. If he did it as nothing more than an ego-enhancing power trip, restraining a willing bottom would hardly serve the purpose. If he did it simply to serve the bottom's interests, there would be little of the Top-bottom power exchange involved and the scene would certainly not be of interest to so many Tops, most of whom despise any overt hint that what they are doing *serves* the bottom. Actually, the key to understanding the Top's interest in a bondage-only scene is among the mysteries of leathersex best understood by doing.

A novice Top is often inspired somewhat by the willingness to provide for a bottom the satisfaction he himself has had as a bottom. He is also moved a bit by the liberty to exercise his newfound power as a Top. No doubt, he is often also motivated by the very question of what a Top gets out of such a scene. Then, having been brought to action by these slight motivations, he feels the almost mystical way that the ropes or other bindings extend his touch, he notices the degree to which the bottom's satisfaction or terror echoes in himself both as the raw emotion it is and as a sense of achievement. Perhaps not the first time he finds himself Topping in a bondage scene, but soon enough, he also discovers the way the rise and fall of the bottom's experience can repeat itself in him if he is vigilant, as he should be, watching out for the bottom's safety and controlling the bottom's experience.

When two people fuck they seldom notice the mechanism which, however rarely, will sometimes raise them both to the pitch of orgasm exactly together. It seems that the same subtle inner devices are at work when the lovemaking is well-done bondage and it appears that these forces are much more easily invoked in bondage than with ordinary fucking. Orgasm is not the point, however, and it almost never actually occurs. What does occur, when everything works perfectly, is an intensification of presence, a powerful experience of well-being, and an overpowering certainty of safety and security.

With all of that always possible, the lesser inspirations suffice. A Top can do a bondage scene because he likes to look at his own handiwork, because he appreciates the resulting sense of power over another person, because his cock responds to the bottom's helplessness, and because he appreciates the extension of his embrace that is represented by the bindings.

What a bottom gets from a bondage scene is not so hard to grasp. In addition to his own version of most everything that accrues for the Top, he also is given the sensations and psychological responses associated with the bondage itself.

There are more styles and types of bondage than can ever be fully enumerated in a book, and each has its own uses, sensations, and effects. The mention of the broadest categories will suggest the possibilities, but the environment, the available equipment, the time constraints, the sexual interests of the men involved, and level of the power exchange between them constantly redefine the options and often encourage innovation.

Leathermen usually speak of bondage by referring to the materials or equipment used.

Rope Bondage

A lot of men who want to do bondage get nervous about rope bondage because they imagine they need to know a lot of fancy knot-tying techniques. Sometimes they feel sure they could get a guy restrained with ropes, but they still worry that their knots and rope patterns will not look good, particularly to the bottom. This is SM stage fright, and it is preposterous.

There is no need for fancy knots in bondage, neither does the pattern of knots and ropes need be handsome or symmetrical. These things may be pleasant, but they are not essential. And, to resolve the problem about the bottom's pleasure with how the bondage looks, it is a simple matter to blindfold him before the tying begins. What is required—and a Top who can't do this ought to find out how before tying anyone up—is the ability to remove the bondage very rapidly in case of emergency.

To make bondage instantly removable, some men learn to make knots that can be released with a simple tug on the exposed rope ends or on specially placed loops. Others keep bolt-cutters within reach, or pruning shears, or other easily used scissors capable of cutting through the rope. And, some of those who do not feel that the purity of a rope bondage would be damaged by it, work out their rope pattern to include steel panic snaps at strategic points. (Panic snaps are discussed in more detail below, in "Chain and Steel Bondage.")

Generally speaking, the point of rope bondage is simple restraint, No particular fantasy scene is suggested by the rope itself. Nonetheless, rope can certainly support all sorts of fantasies: wild west, country boy, historic or modern sailors or pirates, etc.

Just as tying handsome knots is less important than being able to remove the bondage quickly, having the finished web of ropes look good is less important than seeing that it is safe. This is seldom a problem except in the tying of wrists, elbows, and ankles. (See Chapter Seven, "Anatomy, Physiology, and First Aid")

Chain and Steel Bondage

While steel is not a common fetish, it carries with it a lot of the history of punishment and incarceration. It is supercharged with the sounds of clanking, the feel of its icy surface, and the weight with which it hangs on the body. Everything, from handcuffs and steel collars made especially for human restraint to plain chains and snaps found in any hardware store, can be used. And, very commonly, padlocks are worked into chain bondage as well.

Those who enjoy it say that aesthetically pleasing patterns are more easily achieved with chain than with rope. If necessary, it is even possible to count links in the chain to get locks and snaps positioned in perfectly matched pairs. While chains and other steel restraints are less likely than ropes to be installed so tightly that they become dangerous during a scene, they still have to be easily removable. Three major precautions are called for. First, all the locks used in a playroom should be keyed alike, and two copies of the master key should be in the room at all times. If no nearby hardware store sells large sets of keyed-alike locks, go to a locksmith and have him order them. Or ask him to rekey locks he has in stock. This is a normal request for a locksmith to hear and he will not automatically know what you intend to do with them. He probably won't even wonder. Second, bolt cutters sufficient to the task of cutting the chain you are using should also be in the room and easily accessible. It is not necessary that your bolt cutters be adequate to the task of slicing through a super-hardened lock as long as they can handle the chain. Third, at least the most significant of the clips and snaps used should be ones you can easily open. This is where panic snaps are worth their weight in gold, although they are actually very inexpensive.

A panic snap is a steel clip with a specially designed release mechanism, a spring loaded sheath that holds one of the hook ends of the snap in place. It can be released with one hand even when it is bearing the entire weight specified as its load limit (usually thousands of pounds). All you have to do is lift the sheath, and the closed hook falls open. Failure to use panic snaps is an irresponsible act unless you know beyond any shadow of a doubt that you have other equally fast and easy ways of releasing chain bondage.

Even the best steel bondage devices, the ones made very particularly for leathersex applications, are often uncomfortable for the bottom–which may be exactly what you want. The only possible problem with this is that what is a discomfort when the scene begins can become progressive damage by the time the scene is in full swing. While abrasion of the collar bone may be acceptable as an effect of a heavy collar, deep bruising around the atlas vertebra at the base of the skull is not safe since swelling in this area can cause complications involving the spine and will even more easily cause nasty, long-lasting headaches.

Ropes are tailored to fit safely and snugly as they are put in place, handcuffs are adjusted as they are closed, and chains can be tighter or looser by the length of a single link. But ready-made steel restraints are usually not adjustable. Your wonderful, new, steel-strap manacles or collar will not be a one-size-fits-all item. For this reason, and the expense involved in collecting steel bondage devices, it is not unusual for a bottom to come equipped with his own cold, heavy, clanking, steel toys, if that is what it takes to keep him happily restrained.

One note about handcuffs is essential (yes, a warning, another "don't"). Police on television are often seen snapping a closed handcuff against a prisoner's forearm in such a way that the moving half of the cuff is released by the gear teeth, swings away from and under the wrist, and closes by the momentum of the original snap. This is good drama, but it is very bad leathersex. Strains, sprains, fractures, and completely broken bones can result from this flamboyant act. If you have to experiment to understand how it can hurt, even when the force is inadequate to snap the cuffs shut, test your technique on yourself. With a little practice, you can develop moves just as quick and just as professional-looking, but without the dangers. Or, like real police, you can open the cuffs, at least to the last tooth, before pushing them against anyone's arm, then squeeze them as they close. This requires no undue force, but looks great.

Leather and Specialty Bondage

Bondage with leather can mean anything from using thongs and straps of leather as you would cords and ropes, to putting the bottom into one or several leather devices made for restraint. The most common leather bondage items are wrist and ankle restraints. Like short, broad belts, they are very adjustable, often padded or fleece-lined for safety, and usually close with buckles. The buckles can often be padlocked once they are closed.

Many men–Tops and bottoms–are especially fond of leather restraints because they have, to some extent, a leather fetish. Also, odd as it may sound, the capacity to get a bottom in leather bondage using all *matching* restraints is very pleasing, and black leather matches black leather pretty universally. So, a leather hood or head harness, or a blindfold and gag; leather wrist and ankle restraints, or ladders of leather belts made for restraining the legs and arms; a leather bondage belt (fitted with D-rings for attaching rope or chain); and any number of thongs or straps can be used together to produce a handsome, all black, all leather bondage that looks neatly expert, even when installed by a novice.

Cages

A cage or "jail cell" is often found in a well-equipped playroom. The purpose is a sort of bondage, charged with the stuff that fantasies are made of. Whether it is incarceration of a prisoner or keeping an animal out of the way, it is almost impossible to avoid some verbal or mental reference to the fantasies connected with cages when they are used.

Cages can be big enough for the prisoner to pace in, or so confining that your "dog" must curl up tightly to fit in. And, while cages are usually made of bars, they are sometimes more like solid-walled trunks or coffins. When the walls are not bars adequate ventilation is a concern, but an easy one to address.

When the cage is constructed of bars on at least one wall, the imprisoned bottom is still available for torture. If the bars are far enough apart, he may still be available as a cocksucker or urinal as well. A very pleasant way of dealing with a party crowd that has too many bottoms for the number of Tops, is to completely restrain some of the bottoms–in cages if available–and keep them "on tap" for the Tops to take out and use as desired. This method is part of the scene for the right bottoms, and very convenient for roving Tops.

Mummification and Bags

Most kinds of bondage can range from relatively light to extreme in terms of the power exchange, the sensations, and the psychological effects evoked, but mummification is fairly extreme for most players. It is also very popular. The idea of complete mummification is to wrap the bottom, head to toe, in some material that will prevent any movement at all. As the wraps are installed, sensory overloading or sensory deprivation can also be arranged, the degree of breathing can be put in the Top's control, and other devices like catheters or tit clamps might be put in place under or through openings in the wrapping. All these variations carry with them their own safety demands and concerns, but the basic mummy wrap is as easy to learn as it is to enjoy.

Spandex and leather bags are made for the purpose of mummifying bottoms. Elastic and linen bandages, wide latex strips, plastic wrap (the kind used in the kitchen), and tubular knit fabrics are all useful mummy-making materials. Over some of these, layers of duct tape are often applied, producing a solid, shiny, striped surface that invites beating. Anthony F. DeBlase, founder of *DungeonMaster* magazine, teaches mummy-like wrapping of specific body parts to control the degree and type of pain administered and to prevent any blood from getting on whips and clubs. What happens when a mummified body or body part is beaten is that the superficial sting of the whip or rod is reduced, and the deeper, thudding (often bruising) effects of the instrument are increased.

VERBAL ABUSE

Verbal interchange between the Top and the bottom commonly consists of the bottom begging and the Top refusing and delaying, which is good for the power exchange. It also frequently includes the Top degrading the bottom in one way or another, and this is called verbal abuse or verbal humiliation.

Verbal abuse (VA, V/A) sounds like the safest possible leathersex experience. There are no condoms or dental dams required; no ropes or restraints to become overly tight. After all, as everyone knows, "whips and chains may break my skin, but words will never hurt me." Everyone says something like that, but don't you believe it.

Skin's only skin. Stripe it with blazing red welts tonight, and tomorrow (or one day soon) the welts are gone. Their glow may remain in memory, just warm enough to inspire desire, but welts and bruises and even breaks in the skin heal pretty quickly. The surface striped by an out-of-control tongue lashing, on the other hand, doesn't always smooth out and recover so easily.

It is not the place of any book or writer to say that you shouldn't do what gets you off. When it comes to any sex act at all, especially kinky ones, you have to make your own informed choices. With that in mind, there are some things you'll need to know before you start experimenting with verbal scenes.

First, realize that real sex–sex that engages your whole ecstasy-inclined self, regardless of the sex act–is never safe in any absolute way. To be open to deeply satisfying, joyful sex, you have to be vulnerable, not necessarily to germs, but very essentially vulnerable to your partner, soul to soul. This means verbal trips are potential dynamite if you're really *there* for them, really open to the power exchange they express.

Second, recognize your own reasons and reasoning when you're looking for a verbal abuse scene. Top or bottom, you have your reasons. Looking at them does not mean a lot of intense introspection and reflection. That way lies madness, and a lot of bullshit too. Still, look for your own reasoning. Believe your own first impression. It will do for now. Then ask yourself, "Is this about joy, health, fulfillment, and possible ecstasy?" If so, go for it. If not, you may need some form of therapy other than SM play.

Do you want to be called a "filthy cocksucker" because you truly believe that sucking cock makes you (and all gay men?) filthy? If so, will the VA scene feed your self-hatred, or will it help you work through it and deal with it? Your first answer will do. Go with it.

Do you want to be berated because the VA language connects with your early sexual history or with some especially hot porn you treasure in memory? If so, the verbal scene may be nothing more than a way of turning up the sexual heat. Or, it may be a way of beating yourself up for harboring such memories or for no longer being as innocent as you once were. Which is it? Is it okay?

Don't go Freudian. Don't analyze yourself into a corner. Just realize that abusive language can be more scarring than whips and chains. Understand that whether words maim or heal has everything to do with why you enjoy or want them in the first place.

If you decide to experiment with VA, check in with yourself after the scene. Are you recalling the slurs and humiliation as hot, sexy action, or does the memory lead you to doubt your self-worth? Is it a little of each? Even if you decide there does appear to be a dangerous element in VA for you, it is possible to save the sexy side of the action without continuing to put yourself at risk of real damage.

Safety may be as simple as always doing the VA scene as a part of a larger dramatic scene, one in which you *play the part* of the creep or weakling or other worthless slime whose degradation turns you on. Similarly, you may find that there really are things in the realm of leathersex that you don't do well or handle well. Arrange to have your Top degrade you in reference to these acts, keeping you informed outside the scene of your actual progress until such time as the degradation is no longer possible. Get creative. There's always a way to have it all in SM.

The one thing you can't let yourself do is lie to yourself. If you suspect that your reasons for seeking verbal abuse are unhealthy, work that out first. Get all the pain you want, but don't let yourself be harmed.

In a consensual SM scene, VA, like any kind of sex play, has to be within your limits if you're a bottom. Tops, too, can be mentally or emotionally lacerated by the words they sling, so make room for your partner's limits as well. Prepare. Negotiate your verbal scene as carefully as you would a heavy pain trip involving restraint. Then, do what gets you up, what gets you off, and what leaves you high.

PLAYING WITH ANIMALS

To have sex with nonhuman beasts is illegal, frequently dangerous, and not an appropriate subject for leathersex discussion with novices. It can certainly be admitted that sex involving dogs and other animals does take place, but–like sex with children and sex for money–the law is set so squarely against it that even the most evenhanded public discussion is nearly impossible. The legal alternative, which is hotter for most guys anyway, is to reduce your bottom (or be reduced by your Top) to an animal condition.

This doesn't have to be done with dangerous verbal humiliation. It can easily be within the safe fantasy range of most players. In any case, the bottom knows without a doubt that he is a human being, not a dog or work horse, so when the Top gives orders to his dog or horse, he is supporting the fantasy, not hurting the bottom.

The scenes in which the bottom is an animal owned and used by the Top can be extended to any length, including the point of being a recurring part of a relationship, or even its continuing basis. Here, the trappings can be as important as the physical action and verbal elements. Dog bowls, a place to sleep on the floor, mitts that turn hands into paws, and even leg bondage that guarantees the dog will stay on all fours can be great fun. One of the delights of having a dog-boy is that the scene can continue while the Top watches the news on TV, goes out to the market, or otherwise ignores the bottom. Then, too, it can be intensified with training sessions, punishments, and "unwarranted" abuse of the animal which, being only an animal, cannot resist *in human fashion*.

The line between dog and slave sometimes gets very blurred, especially if a dog collar and leash are put on a bottom when the couple go to a bar or party. There is no reason to think that this indistinct role definition is a problem. The Top can let his dog walk upright, or collar his slave like a dog, or leave the question of when the bottom is a slave or an animal entirely unanswered–open to his own moment-to-moment reinterpretation.

STARTING AND ENDING SCENES OF POWER AND SEX

It can sometimes be hard to find the starting point for a scene, the moment at which everyone is in his leathersex role and can let go of the negotiating and "straight time" responsibilities. Winding down and bringing a scene to a clear end can also be difficult. Clumsiness, in getting a scene started or ending it, can ruin the whole experience.

Creativity is often required, especially if the roles for the scene are going to be extreme, and some Tops are especially adept at inventing situations in which a single act or order can move both parties into the exact leathersex mindset required. Other guys stumble and wrestle endlessly with it. If you discover that you are having a problem, one way to get past the discomforts and into the scene is for the two partners to separate for a while, coming back together ready to start the scene immediately. For example, if the intended scene involves the bottom submitting to a flogging, but the conversation before has left the mood too light or friendly for a comfortable transition, the Top can suggest that the bottom go wait—or even go put the restraints on his own wrists and ankles—at the place where the flogging is to take place. After a few minutes, the Top arrives. Either silently or entirely in the role of the flogging Top, he then restrains the bottom or orders him into the right position, and the scene begins.

Another way to get past the clumsiness that can rattle the beginning of a scene is to start out in the mood of the conversation that is underway. If you've been talking about what you want to do, negotiating the scene, and the tenor of the talk has been more interesting than hot, move ahead on interest. "Let's just see if you can really handle that ball stretcher you've been looking at," the Top might say. And the bottom, inching into the scene might either say, "Okay, let's do it," or "Can we give that other toy (whatever it may be) a shot first." The tone is still that of the negotiations, leaving the mood change up to the actual play, a task that leathersex contact is able to handle.

Getting out of the scene can be just as tricky, and ending the scene is made more difficult when it is more important to do it well, as when it is hoped that a night of cuddling and cock sucking will follow. Experienced players usually have less of a problem. In fact, they are almost always able to handle just calling an end to the action at the appropriate moment, and switching directly to hugs and kisses, expressions of their gratitude, immediate departure, or whatever is appropriate. Less experienced players, ones who are likely to need some aftercare or down-loading in order to safely manage the sensory and psychological experience, are the ones who have problems. And seasoned Tops who don't often play with novices sometimes have trouble seeing how to help the novice bottom out of the scene.

What is possible depends very much upon what is needed, but some options can be generalized. One easy way out is to repeat the opening pattern of either a brief separation or a controlled downturn in the mood of the play. These are relatively easy to do if the Top is observant.

It is also relatively easy for leathermen to introduce a final act into a dramatic fantasy either during the negotiation of the scene or by speaking and acting in character at what turns out to be the end. Suppose, for instance, that the fantasy is one in which the foreman is going to sexually abuse a laborer on a construction site. When the Top is finished, he can order the man back to work, perhaps the work of clearing away the toys used in the scene. Alternatively, the bottom can begin to worry aloud about being missed at his job. Whether prearranged or improvised, these ending-moves will work within the scene, permitting it to close naturally.

Whatever else may be going on, if a scene comes to an end for one player, it is not a good idea for his partner to ignore that fact. In a well-prepared scene, the bottom always has recourse to that final, all-stop safe word but, except in scenes meant to test the bottom to his limits, no Top wants to hear that word. To be forced to use that safe word means that the bottom has been pushed to a point where he is, in effect, having to slam on the brakes, a way of stopping at least occasionally as dangerous in the playroom as it is on a wet freeway.

Power games should start and end as naturally as possible, with only as much surprise as is appropriate to the roles of the players in relation to one another. They should proceed within the limits established in negotiations by both parties. And, most importantly, they should leave both or all players feeling good about themselves and the experience they have shared.

Chapter Three

Playing with Pain

The most basic elements of leathersex are the exchange of power between the players, and the intentional stimulation of the bottom by the Top–physically, psychologically, or emotionally. Neither of these is actually the least bit foreign to most adults, regardless of how much they like to profess ignorance. A low-level power exchange is almost essential to satisfying sexual intercourse, and stimulation of one kind or many is absolutely essential. If the stimulation is in the area people commonly call pain, they will either claim to know nothing of its erotic possibilities, or be completely turned off by it. Nonetheless, a great many people who have no interest in leathersex (other than their bias against it) do enjoy the shallow end of the leathersex pool.

Every love-bite or hickey, every nibbled earlobe and every tweaked nipple is directly connected with the pain-seeking and pain-providing instincts of leathersex players. Even tickling and long, hard hugs are related. The point where SM takes over from "normal" sexual play is purely arbitrary.

"I'd like you to slap my butt a little while you fuck me," a trick might say, "but let's not get into any SM. Okay?" A reasonable leathersex player presented with this laughable request keeps his smiles and snickers to himself and accepts the bottom's limits.

People are probably not fooling themselves any better than they are fooling anyone else when they claim to know nothing of pain as erotic stimulation. Still, most people don't do leathersex, and it can certainly be admitted that leathersex is different from "vanilla" sex. Leathersex players approach pain in SM differently than others approach painful sensations during sex. Nevertheless, some of the facts about pain that matter most in the playroom are drawn from very ordinary circumstances, things anyone would understand.

"Pain hurts, but it feels so good when it stops." When I first heard those words, at about age four, I thought my grandfather meant something like: "Won't it be nice when the pain you feel now is all gone and you're 'all better?'" Later, I understood it differently. When posthole digging or fence-wire stringing was getting too painful, he'd say, "Gawn, git to it." Aged eight or nine by then, I'd whine, "But it hurts, Pa!" Then he'd say his famous line: "Pain hurts, but it'll feel so good when it quits. Git with it."

Hours later we'd finish up whatever was the job at hand and, sure enough, I'd find that I had been doing the painfully hard work without feeling any pain. In fact, I was often high on the feeling that had replaced the pain. I couldn't begin to tell you when the pain quit hurting.

Just about everyone must have some experience that can serve as an equivalent to my childhood chores. Sometimes there is pain that you can't run away from–regardless of the reason–which fades away as pain and resurfaces as pleasurable excitement or just a pleasant blank where the unpleasant sensation was. That is the nature of the most common sort of pain leathermen play with, work with, and use in their pursuit of pleasure for themselves and each other.

In recent years, this effect has been explained to some extent by psychopharmacologists and nerve-brain function researchers. The details are all tied up with the release of naturally occurring opiates created in, by, and for the body. Geoff Mains' classic *Urban Aboriginals* covers the subject very well in lay terms, from the point of view of a serious SM player.

You don't really have to read up on the opioids and endorphins, as these biochemicals are called, to use and enjoy them. But, this is the first principle of pain as sexual pleasure that every leatherman has to understand, even if the understanding is always entirely tacit or even unconscious: The pain we are dealing in, except in special or extreme cases, is pain as a means, not an end. It is pain as a method to intensify sensation and as a route to pleasure, even as access to ecstasy. Often, it might be said, leathermen give and take pain as a means of achieving an "endorphin high." It is pain as a safe recreational drug; not pain as pointless suffering.

Without getting lost in the labyrinthine possibilities of the subject by trying to explain every variation, exception, and permutation, we can move on to the second principle: limits. The degrees of pain a person is willing to withstand in conjunction with various activities—basically, while waiting for it to quit hurting—are called his "limits," and they are important barriers. If they are crossed, meaning that the Top is providing more stimulation or more intense stimulation than the bottom is willing or able to bear, any and all pain is likely to become focused, terrible, plain, pointless agony.

So, the establishment of limits is of paramount importance to a novice. Ensuring that the Top you go home with can be trusted to respect your limits, and assuring yourself that he understands what those limits are, can be vitally important too. On the other hand, having limits that are too restrictive or too timid can mean that you will never experience the liberating pleasures that make masochism the irresistible sex-style it is for uncounted millions.

You want the experience that leathersex represents, but you don't want to "go too fast." You want to give a Top the opportunity to "take you further than you have ever gone," but you don't want to end up seriously injured. And, although you may never before have thought of it, you don't want your limits to be so restrictive or to change so slowly that nothing happens . . . ever. If you always keep your pain-acceptance limits at the threshold of your existing ability to "bear" the hurt, the limit will progress but you will not. You will find yourself inviting and taking more pain without moving a single inch closer to ecstasy.

The ecstatic in leathersex is approached only by leaps. You have to overstep your supposed limits by giant steps to get there. If the limit just creeps up, you are effectively building up a psychic callous rather than moving toward the ecstatic leap. For this reason—and other obvious reasons like safety—you want to put yourself into the hands of Tops you trust *completely*. Then you will relax your limits more, take greater apparent risks, and, in the end, risk ecstasy more than injury. But this is true only if the Top is actually experienced and knowledgeable and the trust is flawless (up to the point that it is tested).

All of which adds up to one imperative for the novice in leathersex: Set your limits always beyond what you imagine them to be, but test your limits only with a Top you trust to know your body better than you know it yourself. Doing this, the thing you will be risking more than anything else is that you might possibly pass out of ordinary experience into the intensity that makes leathersex the marvel that it is.

The following sections examine some of the ways leathermen play with pain.

STARTING POINTS

A man who never suspected he had any leathersex inclination can discover a great deal about himself when, out of the blue, his sex partner claps an open hand against exposed skin. If the first flush of surprise brings with it a sense of humiliation and a thrill, an urge to submit and a willingness to do so, an impish inclination to fight back, or a determined will to retaliate, the information is telling. Beyond pleasure-in-pain, what you're likely to discover the first time someone plants a hand print on your ass is the very basis of your leathersex orientation.

Then, for most people, some variation on that first slap and their reaction to it becomes an essential part of their leathersex repertoire. It can be spanking, flogging, or whipping. It can involve belts, paddles, hands, crops, quirts, or just about anything. It can be done in the context of just about any fantasy, under any set of partner-defining labels, and it can be anything from a ritualized suggestion to an outright beating. Still, pain produced by blows is surely the most nearly universal physical element in SM, and in those degrees of leathersex that the participants would not call SM as well. And, no instruments of pain are more commonly used than the hands themselves.

Many novices in leathersex discover that in any individual scene the first blow serves the purpose of helping them to discover just how they want to relate to their partner of the moment. Later, with more experience to rely on, men make more reasoned choices about what to do and how to respond. Experience develops the resources needed to ignore, for example, an overly eager first blow in favor of a Top's good reputation. While waiting for the benefits of experience to accrue, a bottom has little other than his response to the first blow or two to work with as he determines how to settle into (or refuse) a scene. From timidly receptive to hungrily demanding, a bottom's reactions in the first moments of a scene are messages to himself about his role in the scene at hand.

The important thing to bring into your understanding of coming to erotic blows is the persistent theme of all leathersex: safe, sane, consensual activity. Let's start with the question of consent. If you are the bottom, meaning you are the one who will be receiving the blows and expecting erotic pleasure from them or in connection with them, it is vitally important that you communicate the exact extent of your consent to the Top.

The best advice for a novice is that you start by consenting to hands only, and that you consent to nothing without knowing that you are able to stop the scene if it goes further than you are ready to go. Within a single scene, you may find yourself ready to extend your consent to paddles, cats-o'-nine, belts or whatever, as a product of trust developed within the power exchange. And, for scenes involving restraints, bondage, or whipping toys that can break the skin, it is probably best to refuse altogether until you know the Top and the situation well. You might, for instance, hold out (especially on scenes involving whips) until you have seen the Top in action with another bottom.

As to the safety and sanity of scenes involving spanking and whipping, normal cautions apply, with the added reminder that a man who is perfectly trustworthy in all other situations can become hyperstimulated by the physical acts and the resulting sounds of these scenes. Don't lose your own responsible judgement (or, for that matter, become too cautious), and don't let the scene carry your partner away. This danger exists in all leathersex scenes, but is heightened in the atmosphere of spanking and whipping, particularly for novices. Get off on it. Let yourself go. But keep your wits about you, too.

One of the great charms of spanking and whipping–an essential pleasure for some of us–is the marking of the flesh. It can have both immediate effects and more lasting pleasures, but this too is a matter of negotiated limits. Are you willing to have welts and marks? Are you only willing to have marks for the duration of the scene, for the night, for a few days? Do you expect that if a break in your skin appears the Top should immediately stop the scene? Do you want deep pains that might be restarted over several days when you sit or shower, or only surface stimulation? Know what you want, how much more than that (if any) you are willing to accept, and how to talk to your partner about it.

Finally, the question of safe and sane "beating" involves a certain amount of information that ought to be intentionally learned in some other way than by trial and error. For this there are two options, and the best route is to take *both*. First, there are instructional classes, books, and videos available. Don't mistake erotic fiction in print or on video for instruction. Some of the acts described with loving care in fiction are not safe, some are not even possible. Even what you see on video, or believe you see, may not be what is actually happening. Instructional media identifies itself as such, and even then needs to be judged on its inherent merits rather than its claims about itself. Second, there is learning by watching others who already have experience, which is a perfectly good excuse for going to leather events where there will be demonstrations and to SM play parties, too.

SPANKING, SPECIFICALLY

Spanking is a major theme in leathersex, especially among novices. For some guys, in fact, spanking is the one act beyond ordinary oral and anal sex that interests them. It can be explained to death with reference to how kids are punished or not, how kids thought they ought to have been punished or not, and any number of other psychological and sociological factors, but none of that works. The more spanking fans you know, the more mutually exclusive explanations you will also get to know. The only constant is that spankers and the bottoms they play with do it because they enjoy it.

Taking spanking to mean hitting with an open hand, it is obvious that the prime targets will be the ass and the face. The former is about a thousand times safer a striking zone than the latter, but every player works out his own levels of acceptable risk based on his own experience of desire and pleasure. Certainly there are also guys who get off on having their backs, chests, thighs, and the bottoms of their feet slapped. And there are plenty of guys who are more than happy to oblige them, too.

There are, for some players, elements of humiliation in any kind of spanking, especially ass beatings and face slappings. But humiliation is not necessarily part of it. There are elements of role playing in a lot of spanking scenes–from the correcting coach and his poorly performing student, to the bad boy and his dad. Again, roles are not necessarily part of the scene.

What is essential to a spanking scene is the hand hitting the bottoms's body repeatedly. That alone does the trick for a lot of guys, and its naturally connected variations–like gripping and squeezing the spanked skin, rubbing the area soothingly or roughly–are all part of the spanking.

What can be done with an open hand can also be done with a paddle. The thing that sets paddles apart from other leathersex toys is that they are designed to make contact with a fairly large area of the body with each blow, like open hands only more so. This spreads the stimulation out a bit and gives the type of pain experienced in a hand or paddle spanking a different range of sensations than other instruments are likely to provide. Paddles also give the spanker a chance to rest his hand, which can become as spanked as the bottom's bottom in some scenes. Besides, paddles come in all sizes and shapes, materials and weights, providing a nearly infinite array of possible experiences for the connoisseur.

Spanking, whether with hands or paddles, is about the safest kind of pain-related leathersex. Of course, hands or paddles applied indiscriminately and heavily to the area of the kidneys, to the gut or lower back, or to the neck and other joints can be dangerous, but slaps in these areas are hardly erotic for most people anyway.

Spanking in one form or another plays an important role in the sexual fantasies and erotic lives of many people who do not think of themselves as leather folk at all. They advertise in personal ads that they miss the spankings Dad used to give them. They order spanking videos and place themselves vicariously in the role of the bottoms as they watch the tapes over and over. Or, they swat the asses of the men they're with, in the hope of getting a few "good ones" in return.

Since spanking is the most common facade behind which undeveloped SM interests hide, it is especially important to question yourself if you find yourself saying, "I'm not into SM, I just like to be spanked." It could be true, but likely not. Push the question harder if you find that you are all the more interested when the spanker is willing to shift from his open hand against your ass to a paddle, belt, or cane.

On the other hand, it is actually possible that there are people who don't want to experience the full leathersex power exchange, people who just want their butts whacked soundly from time to time. Anything is possible.

CANES AND RODS

This category of toys runs the gamut from nearly harmless bamboo sticks that break under fairly light use to heavy riot batons that can easily crush bones. The possible fantasy scenes vary widely with the history and appearance of the instrument, from English schoolboy punishments to brutal cops on the rampage. As the density of the material increases from hollow bamboo upward, and the size of the instrument increases from under a quarter of an inch to more than two inches in diameter, the possibility of inflicting real damage increases proportionately.

Nonetheless, in even moderately experienced hands, a cane is a relatively safe toy, particularly when the scene calls for it to be used on the ass (lots of muscle for padding) or in a boy's school style punishment (few and counted strokes). Spanking is one natural precursor to caning, with the Top sometimes suggesting a cane in order to save his hands while still delivering as much pain and punishment as the bottom wants.

Knowing something of the geography of the body is more important with canes and rods than it is with an open hand, but what is needed is easily learned (see Chapter Seven, "Anatomy, Physiology, and First Aid"). Besides, if the Top starts off relatively gently and is watching at all, the bottom's reactions will give him a reliable map of the pleasure, pain-pleasure, and dangerous pain zones.

Striking any area of the body once with a cane provides a certain sort of sensation—usually more sting with narrower instruments, a more deeply felt thud with a thicker one. Striking many times in the same general area gives a different kind of sensation, especially as the lines of the strokes cross or coincide with one another. What was stinging tends to become an even sharper kind of pain until the area becomes evenly reddened (called "leathered up"), at which point the pain spreads quickly and changes character dramatically, although the direction of change is different for different people.

Striking the very same spot repeatedly with a narrow instrument, however, is another matter altogether. This is torture, pure and simple. The sting of a cane pounding over and over in the same spot grows in depth and intensity, even though the strokes are not becoming harder at all, until the pain is excruciating. It is impossible to believe that a tiny little dowel or bamboo stick can be the vehicle of such powerful pain, but it can. Instead of welts and stripes, this use of a cane will leave long-term bruises, and often leaves the area sore for days or even weeks, a handsome reminder of a Top's long and careful attention to a single stripe or even one square inch of your thigh or butt.

As the rods get thicker, the same energy put into each stroke obviously delivers a greater blow to the bottom, and brings with it a greater demand for the Top to know what he is doing. A lead shot-loaded riot baton, or a short length of heavy rubber hose, for example, can easily break bones.

Broken bones may be acceptable to some bottoms, but they go against the grain of the leathersex version of the law of the conservation of matter and energy. That law, in its simplest form says: Bottoms should always be used and abused with an eye to their recyclable nature. That is, a good bottom should be handled in such a way that an infinite number of Tops might also use the same bottom an indeterminate number of times in the future. Not breaking the bottom is half the job of following this rule. The other half is leaving the bottom ready for more. If he isn't ready to go again immediately, a well-used bottom should still be eager to get more when he can.

Thicker rods, police batons particularly, are also good oral and anal dildoes. (Condoms and proper cleaning should be used, of course.) The connection of sexual penetration and the instrument with which the bottom is being beaten can be a great turn-on for Top and bottom. Of course the same connection can be made by sticking your hand into a bottom's mouth or ass, but nothing of the sort is possible with narrow canes and rods. The dangers to the mouth and throat are tremendous. Why else would your mother and your teachers have been so upset every time they caught you daydreaming, with a pencil sliding in and out of your mouth? And inserting something as stiff and narrow as a cane into a guy's asshole is really unthinkable. The injuries can range from annoying cuts and abrasions at the rectal opening to life-threatening tears and punctures of the intestines.

While it is possible to play interactive games with just about any striking instruments in the dungeon, rods and canes provide especially fun options for counting games. "Your bad behavior has earned you six of the best with this cane. Count them off, and be grateful for the correction." To which the bottom answers, "Yes, Sir," and counts, "One, Sir. Thank you, Sir. May I have another?" By the time we get to "Six, Sir. Thank you, Sir," there will surely have been a count that was not worded perfectly (a separate opportunity for punishment), or a count that was too muffled to be heard clearly (an opportunity to repeat the stroke and get it clearly counted). Besides, a boy can always be punished for taking his punishment too bravely–the sin of pride, obviously.

If your idea of leathersex includes being restrained while you are punished, rods and canes are probably going to be more to your liking than a man's hand. The length of the rod and the need to have space to swing it often set the Top apart from the bottom a bit, leaving room for dungeon furniture you can be tied to (a whipping post, a caning bench, etc.). Bondage sometimes also seems to get in the way of the fantasies that are common in bare-handed spanking (the woodshed, Dad sitting on the foot of your bed, etc.), but fits right in with the roles most likely to succeed where canes and rods are used (POW, police interrogation, etc.).

Except when they are recurring parts of a scene involving any number of *other* leathersex activities, rods and canes tend to be used in relatively short scenes. Spanking scenes might be up to 30 minutes each and repeated several times in an evening. Floggings can go on for several hours and often do. But, a serious caning that runs to more than 20 strokes is uncommon. Then, obviously, there are the die-hard fans–Top and bottom–who can do whatever it is for as long as the other guy lasts.

FLOGGERS AND WHIPS

Flogging, lashing, and whipping. Cat-o'-nine tails, bullwhip, black snake, and dog quirt. Words like these–and Whip-master–seem to be at the center of the modern conception of sadomasochism. That may be as it should, yet they convey for most people images of the most extreme violence, and they are attached to a realm of activity that most people cannot consider even remotely safe or sane, an area where they would argue that any consent to participate is merely a symptom of deep-rooted illness.

Who cares? People may think what they will, flogging is fun. It might be the most common physical SM activity where two or more can play, but each truly successful flogging is its own kind of rare and wonderful experience.

If you have never been flogged, what do you imagine it might be like? Whatever your answer, you can be as right or wrong as you choose. Depending on the whip and force used and on the skill of the Top, a flogging can be anything from a gentle, massage-like form of lovemaking to a monstrous, flesh-tearing pain scene. And, despite the fact that most novices seem to have developed a fear of whips before they even see one, a good flogging by a good Top under the right conditions is an excellent introduction to the world of SM.

With a trusted and experienced Top who knows you are new to SM, you can negotiate a scene that is required to begin with gentle strokes from a soft, caressing whip, then progress at *your* pace to heavier strokes and heavier whips.

Here's what to look for when you first get to taste the loving lash: Look for the difference between stinging, superficial sensations, and thudding sensations that are felt deeper in the tissues. When you can notice the difference–which is very easily done–think about which you like better and why. Look for the way the sensations are different on your shoulders, the broad part of your back, your ass, and wherever else you may be stroked. Think about where you like the whip to land, and why that is better for you. Look for a correlation between the sounds, if any, and the sensations. Decide whether this is a significant part of the trip for you, how, and why. Now, be willing to talk about these things to the man who helped you sample them.

It is important that you discuss your early experience specifically with the same Top you played with because he will know things about his own whips that no one else will know. He will, for instance, be able to notice if the floggers you like are deerskin or kangaroo, rather than cowhide. He will notice from what you say whether you are a fan of the instruments he tends to use most heavily or lightly, in broader or more concentrated areas. And, having watched your reactions, he will be able to help you sort out the difference between your struggle to relax and your actual responses to the flogging.

Of course, it might as well be admitted that not everyone will be able to find, in walking distance of home, a patient and kindly Top with a large whip collection. What then? Improvise with a friend. Get belts, long leather thongs of various thicknesses and weights, a few lengths of rubber tubing (not heavy rubber hose for this experiment), and maybe some thick, round electric cords (lamp cord, the usual weight of household extension cords is hard to handle and easily breaks skin). You're probably going to get high, hard, and horny from this little experiment, so do it with someone you wouldn't mind fucking with a little later in the program.

Instructions for the stand-in Top: Have your novice bottom lie down on the floor, face down, with his forearms under his face. This is a multi-prong safety posture useful because you are both beginners. Then, with each belt or bundle of thongs, tubes, or cords, toss the first few strokes into the air and let them land on nothing but their own weight on the novice bottom's back or ass. (His choice, why not?) Remembering that you are using improvised substitutes for floggers, things that are likely to be unruly or worse, do this toss-and-fall stroke several times to get an idea how the "whip" works before you begin to actually swing, adding force and direction of your own. Then work up very slowly. (You might even lay the first strokes at each new intensity on a pillow or the edge of a bed, just to see how they go.) Think in terms of no more than thirty minutes overall time for the in-action portion of the experiment. Hold open the possibility of taking and giving additional tastes of specific instruments a bit later.

Try not to hit in such a way that any part of any instrument falls on the bottom's neck or head. Since we're aiming for pleasure, try to stick to the muscles, away from the lower back and spine. Use sweeping, side-to-side strokes to strike the ass, and single direction, shoulder-to-waist strokes for the back. If you see reddened lines appearing, don't worry. Keep working in the same areas, spreading slightly, but not extending to the neck, lower back, or legs. Soon, you should notice that the redness is less a pattern of lines, more a generally colored area. This is completely normal. The skin, as it is said, has leathered up. It is now both more sensitive and, very likely, more receptive to additional strokes.

After a while, always adjusting your force, direction, and instrument to suit the bottom's experimental needs, stop and make time to talk about the sensations. Well, no, as a matter of fact, it wouldn't hurt to fuck first and talk later, but not a whole lot later.

If you can find some real whips, that only makes the taste test that much easier and that much more usefully conclusive. And, if you can also arrange to have an experienced Top play the role of the Top in your experiment, so much the better.

So, just in case you find yourself in a city with a decent toy store, it wouldn't hurt for you to have some idea of what sorts of whips to look for. On the other hand, the very best whips are not likely to be found in even the best leather toy stores, although anything can happen these days. Here is what we might call a far from cheap, nonetheless very basic whip collection: A horsehair "swish" or flyswatter; a lightweight, soft leather flogger with no fewer than 18 flat, nonbraided tails; a medium to heavy flogger, probably with more flat tails, definitely made of heavier leather. Already, your collection is going to serve you well in most social and fantasy scenes. For the next advance, you may want a braided flogger, usually a cat-o'-nine tails, with either small knots or flat tags at the ends of the tails. And, finally, for the adventurous, a single-tailed whip of some kind is next. A signal whip, with the cracker removed, is a good place to start with single-tailed whips.

There you are, five whips that make up an extremely versatile arsenal. If you're thinking something like, "I'm the bottom; I don't need to own whips," you may be a bit out of step with the times. These days, probably with little reason to be so concerned, a lot of guys have the idea that whips (like uncleaned dildoes and IV needles) are one-man toys. So, in some areas of the country, and in some clubs, the rule seems to be that if you want a flogging, you provide the instruments of your own stimulation.

A special note on single-tailed whips: These whips, with a thin strip of rawhide or nylon, the cracker, attached at the end, are not made for striking anyone. They aren't even made for striking cattle and other thick-skinned beasts. When it cracks, the tip of the whip is actually breaking the sound barrier, and you don't want anything moving that fast to touch your skin. It would slice through like a knife. Properly used, a bullwhip or black snake, cracker and all, is meant to produce a noise that moves animals by frightening them. While there are a few whipmasters able to turn a long whip into a remarkable SM experience, the proper man-to-man use of such whips requires long and careful training for the Top, and absolute trust from the bottom. All the same, a relatively short single-tailed whip, like a signal whip or target whip, with the cracker removed, can certainly be used for striking and striping human skin.

In a later chapter, you will find basic physiological information that will help you decide where to whip and be whipped, but generally, light enough whips, used lightly enough, can be applied anywhere except the face. Heavier whips and heavier strokes should be applied where they fall on muscle rather than bones or joints. For areas where a lot of control is called for, like the genitals, special whips are also called for. And, the basic principle that rules everything else is that the Top must know what he is doing, exactly what he is doing, and how it is affecting you.

Flogging is a sensual delight for Top and bottom whether it is done in a brutal punishment mode or a sweet and loving style, but it only works when the guy running the physical show, the Top, cares about doing it right. If he cares, he'll find out what right means. If he doesn't care, fire him. No matter how many times you hear that good Tops are hard to find, a bad Top is never an acceptable substitute.

CREATIVE PLAYTHINGS FOR LEATHERSEX

One of the great pitfalls of leathersex is the uncontrollable urge to collect dungeon toys. There seems to be no cure for it and, except for impending bankruptcy, little reason to wish for a cure. Every new toy is a new excuse to play again with occasional partners.

Every new toy leads to new and often interesting ways of producing variations on the established sensation themes.

Some collectors only want toys they can use, while others want historic instruments regardless of whether they can still be used safely. Others are looking for instruments of real torture, the sort used by The Inquisition, that are designed to do permanent damage. While very few historic torture implements have a place in leathersex, some are great dungeon decorator items, and replicas are sometimes available in museum shops. Real or replicated, examine these things carefully before deciding to use them. Apart from being built to damage, some of the replicas are so flimsy they can cause unexpected injuries just by falling apart at the wrong time.

Modern torture instruments, however, made by leathermen who *adapt* the scary, old-time devices, can be great fun. They carry along with them all the bone-chilling history of POW tortures, The Inquisition, or whatever their origin suggests, but are adjusted for the age of the recyclable bottom.

Another category of toys that has been around for a very long time might be called "toys pressed into service." Red-figure cups from fifth century BC Athens show sandals and slippers being used as paddles for beating ass. The idea was good then and works just as well today, 2,500 years later. Of course belts are popular for ass beating and can be used even for striking the chest and back, as they have been for at least several centuries. Similarly, clothespins were not originated for leathersex use, much as it may seem that there is little other reason for their continued sale in cities where no one ever hangs laundry out to dry.

Many other household items are pressed into leathersex service on a regular basis–chopsticks, large spoons and spatulas, and the clamps used to close potato chip bags, for instance. So are medical devices like sutures, clamps, hemostats, and elastic bandages, and items made for farm and veterinary use such as hobbles, castrating bands, and electric prods. Pet supplies, tools, hardware store standards, and restaurant equipment are also used. A large rubber spatula–a giant version of the wooden-handled kind used to scrape mixing bowls–makes a marvelous, high-density paddle, for instance, but the rubber and wood have to be glued together to withstand the centrifugal force of a high-speed swing. And there is the warning you must bear in mind as you select items from the kitchen, hardware store, pet shop, or feed supply store for your leathersex use. Many of them will require careful testing under safe conditions, most will require some slight modification, and all will be deficient in some ways. The above-mentioned rubber spatula needed to have a powerful glue stuffed into the rubber socket to keep the wooden handle in place, *and* it is hard to get it as clean as you might like it to be.

The idea of pressing ordinary objects–called "pervertibles" by New York writer David Stein–into dungeon service is intriguing. It can be fun, and it can add both variety and humor to your play time. And, while it must be done with great care, it can sometimes be a lifesaver. Imagine yourself on a business trip without your toy bag. Suppose you meet the leatherman of your dreams on the convention floor. He says he'll be at your hotel room at, say, 7:00. What to do? No problem. Hotel rooms and hotel gift shops are bulging with leathersex paraphernalia, once you get your imagination running in that groove.

The little clotheslines and clothespins they sell in the gift shop, usually labelled as though they were for drying panty hose and lingerie only, are useful for both bondage and pain trips. Washcloth gags and hand towel blindfolds work superbly. Sometimes the shower curtain rod is a heavy pipe set deep into two solid walls, providing the needed crossbar portion of a whipping cross. The firm, square-edged hotel mattress, pulled out of alignment with the box springs, provides a split level arrangement that can be a perfectly acceptable substitute for a sling. And there is a lot more you can do, depending on what you find in the room, what you happened to have in your luggage (shaving scene, anyone?), and what you can pick up without leaving the hotel. Obviously, not every scene can be put together perfectly on a moment's notice in a hotel room, but if the limitations of the location preclude or destroy the scene, it probably has as much to do with failed chemistry between you and your man as with anything else. After all, he will arrive with his hands, belt, shoes, socks, and underwear, and he will find yours there as well.

It is often said in leathersex circles that the most important sex organ a leatherman has is his brain. This is true because we play with fantasies and ideas, because we play with terror and appearances, and also because we often have to get very creative with the items in our environment to provide ourselves with the basics of leather action.

ABRASION

The very mention of abrasion as erotic activity will set vanilla guys to squirming. In fact, a good many leathermen shudder when they first hear of it, but the more they learn of it, the more likely that they will find at least one form of abrasion that suits them comfortably. We aren't talking about tearing away whole muscles with an electric sander, of course. On the contrary, erotic abrasion is usually a tiny, delicate sort of stimulation.

Like many aspects of leathersex, abrasion is something most people will claim to know nothing about, but they do. You do. Whether you like it or not, someone–intending seduction or expressing passion–has raked his fingernails down your spine, or trailed them across your chest. That's it. Abrasion, like so many aspects of sexual behavior, is an instance where leathersex just takes the ordinary action and amplifies it, elevating the thrill of a moment into the ecstatic experience of the evening, perhaps–you never know–of a lifetime. The difference is that in leathersex, to perform Sex Magic rather than settling for the momentary sparkle, some toys are often called for.

Emery boards and vegetable brushes, pot scrubbers and sandpaper, chain mail butcher's gloves and rubber-studded construction gloves are good abrasion toys. And, just as with many other categories of play, once you get going, you'll find lots of ready-made household items lying around–pervertibles–just waiting to be used.

Nipples respond nicely to light abrasion, and even better to full-on bloodletting if the bottom is up to it. Cock heads, the coronal ridge of the cock, the shaft of the cock, the scrotum, and the perianal area are each separate abrasion playgrounds where you will get very different results with quite similar amounts of rubbing. It isn't unheard of to have abrasive techniques used on any and all body parts, but some areas probably ought to be considered off-limits. The face and tongue, for instance, are not erotic zones when it comes to abrasion. Although, that said, there will now be experimenters who will decide nothing is sexier than having their tongues and faces sanded raw. While it is possible and even pleasant to abrade the asshole and the first inch or two inside (rubber-studded gloves are perfect for starting this, emery boards would be more advanced), it is not a good idea to use any abrasive technique in the urethra (inside the cock). The possibility of infection is extremely high, and even uninfected healing can cause deformities of the dick.

Light abrasion can feel like it is tearing away tissue long before the skin breaks at all. This is enough of a trip for some people, and can be quite intense with the appropriately terrorizing atmosphere, bondage, blindfolds, the Top's "reactions" to the scene, etc. Slightly heavier or longer abrasion, or abrasion performed with sharper toys (like a nutmeg grater), will lead rather quickly to clear fluids weeping out through the skin, with actual bleeding following soon. Heavy abrasion, which should always be worked up to slowly, does just what it feels like it is doing. It tears away layers of skin and lets the blood flow out of surface capillaries.

Obviously, bleeding is only a problem if it is a problem for one of the parties involved. For safety's sake, clean or sterile conditions will be required to protect the bottom from infection once the skin is broken. If toys that have drawn blood, even tiny amounts of blood, are not to be discarded after the scene, they must be objects that can be thoroughly cleaned. Then, of course, they must be thoroughly cleaned before they are reused.

The very special allure of abrasion is that it is a good, quiet, not terribly strenuous way for a Top to spend a few hours giving his undivided attention to a bottom, an almost meditative scene. It makes a good combination with mummification if the Top simply doesn't wrap, or carefully removes the wrappings from, the body parts he wants to sand.

STRETCHING

Unlike abrasion, stretching is usually done on a relatively large scale. Most commonly, the balls are drawn to the bottom of the scrotum, bound or wrapped, then pulled or weighted. If this is done slowly enough, under the right conditions, the extent to which even a novice's balls can be separated from his body both safely and enjoyably is remarkable. The right conditions, as any man would guess, include warmth to keep the balls loose, whatever sound the bottom has been trained to find soothing (his Master's voice?), and a steady, confident installation of the wrappings or ball stretcher. Fiddling with the balls a lot trying to get a stretcher wrapped around them just makes it harder and harder to get the thing on. If there's already been a bit of fumbling, in fact, the stretcher will be on sooner if you just stop, relax a bit, and start over.

Nipples can be stretched rather impressively too. If they are pierced, it is better to stretch them by putting a piece of sturdy cord or string around the nipple so it runs up or down behind both sides of the jewelry. If not, a snake bite kit, vacuum pump, or elastrators can be used to beef up the buds to the point where a short length of cord can be tied around each nipple. Then this tied-around cord can be used as the blocking mechanism to keep your stretching instruments–fingernails, another cord, or whatever–from slipping off.

Stretching the whole body on a rack is also pleasant, but the number of racks available in any given neighborhood is fairly small, so you may not get to use one every day. Because body stretching puts significant stresses on joints, muscles, and even the spine, it is essential that you learn exactly what is safe and what is dangerous before getting serious about using a rack. Do not depend on the bottom's reactions or verbal cues to keep the scene safe. It is not unusual for a person being stretched on a rack to feel that all is not just well, but entirely perfect, only to discover a dislocated joint when the pressure comes off, or unexpected aches and bruises the next morning.

Some enjoyable variations on the stretching of accessible body parts such as balls and nipples are easily discovered. The cords used for stretching can be threaded through a small pulley on the ceiling above the bench or bed. Then you can play with the cords yourself, hang weights from them, or both. Since the joy of being stretched is cumulative–meaning that it becomes tolerable, then comfortable, and only later thrilling, and delicious–a wise Top will find something else to do while the bottom swims up through the stages of pleasure. A good time for some of that abrasion, no?

CLOTHESPINS, CLAMPS, AND PINCHING

Most guys get a lot of their earliest SM by playing with themselves, just as they got most of their first sexual strokes that way.
Among the easiest leathersex toys to discover, get a supply of, and
play with are clothespins and other clamps. So, naturally enough,
clothespins and clamps are popular first-pain-scene toys. Besides,
Mom and Pop may be shocked if they discover a dresser drawer full
of dildoes, floggers, or piercing equipment, but a few clothespins,
woodworker's clamps, or even medical clamps can be explained
away pretty convincingly, especially if they were never quite *hidden* anyway.

In those first halting steps toward leathersex stardom, a lot of
guys put clothespins–usually not all that many at any one time–on
just about all the same body parts experienced players put them on.
After all, SM play styles are nothing more than an accumulation of
the discoveries of individual people. What works gets done; what
gets done spreads and is repeated.

Where, for instance? Nipples are usually discovered right away,
but the more adventurous start right off with their own cock and
balls. Foreskins droop under the weight of four, five, six, or more
wooden clothespins. The scrotum can be turned into a porcupine-
like ball of clothespin spines. The shaft of the cock can sustain at
least one solid row of pins, two if the first row doesn't pinch up too
much of the loose skin. The ears, nasal septum, armpits, lips,
tongue, eyebrows, the ridge between the balls and the asshole, and
even the rim of the asshole are often early discoveries as well. All of
these are fun places for a Top to place the pins on a bottom too. Just
because you can do it yourself is no reason to prefer doing it yourself. (You can make yourself come, too, but you wouldn't want to
restrict that to parties of one only. Would you?)

You really can't put a row of clothespins or any similar clamps
down each side of your own spine either, but there are other reasons to explore this kind of pain-pleasure with someone else. The
excitement of the power exchange between a Top and a bottom
during a lengthy clothespin scene can be incredible. There is
something intensely intimate about a kind of action that puts the
interplay on such an obvious stroke-by-stroke basis. Another pin

here? Another pin at all? If unspoken, these questions still reverberate constantly in both the Top and the bottom after the scene gets well underway.

The nature of clamping as torture is very special too. It may hurt or not to put a clamp in place, depending where it is placed, with what force it closes, and how many other treatments that body area has already had. Soon enough, though, almost all clamp placements stop hurting. They contribute to the sensations you are working with and getting high on, but they are not identified as pain sites. Each clamp can remain comfortable this way for a long time, eventually even arriving at a numb or no-sensation state. How soothing. If the Top toys with the clothespins, wiggling or slapping them, there is some sensation, sometimes even some pain in the *surrounding* tissues. But generally, the numbness and the pleasant sense of accomplishment are with you as long as the clamps are. How nice. Watch out. Sooner or later the pressure has to come off. When it does, blood will rush in where no blood has been able to go, and the fireworks can be spectacular.

One delicious sort of clothespin/clamp scene is this: You put two or three hundred clothespins on a guy's body, saving stripes down the front of his body for last, preferably stripes that run across his nipples, converging in his pubic hair. Then, instead of placing separate clothespins along these reserved stripes, you install "zippers," clothespins strung together like beads on a cord or leather thong. Then, when it is time to remove the pins you make a fuss about the need to get them off before the clamped tissues reach the point that the pain of having the pins taken off will be too intense for the bottom. (This can be true enough, by the way.) Last on, last off, so the zippers are still in place when all the other pins are gone. Instead of unclipping the pins on the zippers, you could just rip them off all at once. That is nice, but nowhere near the limit of screaming super-sensation possible. Instead, keep the bottom occupied for a while–fuck him silly, flog him, do whatever it takes to keep him distracted–zippers bouncing and wriggling in place. Then tie the ends of the zippers to something and tell the bottom he had better get those clothespins off soon. Already the pain is going to be astounding. What will it be like if he leaves them on still longer? And, to get them off, he will have to back away from whatever he is tied to. No problem: Man against a few clothespins. At this point, you stand back and watch the struggle as your bottom tries to defer pain, knowing he's storing up worse pains for himself in the process. Sweet. (And there are people who don't even understand sadism, much less enjoy it!)

There are not a lot of warnings required for clothespins, but you want to be very careful in choosing other kinds of clamps. Still, the rule is simple enough, and absolutely effective: Don't put a clamp on anyone until you know from personal experience precisely what kind of sensation the clamp produces on the very body part you are planning to clamp. Tops who can't take at least a little test squeeze from a clamp have no right to go sticking it on bottoms to find out what happens.

Variations on the straight clothespins on/clothespins off scene primarily have to do with how they are taken off. They can be popped off with a signal whip, one by one. They can be roughly flogged off, by handfuls even. They can be wrestled off, exercised off, or removed by having the bottom stretch himself this way and that until, without touching them, he is able to make every pin snap off his skin. All of these methods, and the many others that are already known or soon to be discovered, require that the Top know what works and what doesn't, what is possible and what is not. For example, clothespins and clamps placed on the forearms cannot necessarily be removed by the bottom wriggling and stretching and not touching them. This is not necessarily a reason for failing to order him to do so. Anything may be fair, depending on the scene and the relationship, but the Top who *doesn't know* just wrecks everything for everyone.

SPOT TORTURE

A lot of men who are interested in leathersex are uncomfortable with the idea of being restrained, being tied down in such a way that they might not be able to change their situation if they wanted to. And, of course, a lot of novices are uneasy about their limits with regard to tolerating pain. One way of dealing with these discomforts, and finding whole new realms of pleasure at the same time, is to explore spot bondage and spot torture.

It is even possible to ease into leathersex with the man of your choice by limiting the nonvanilla exposure to just a designated body part. Cock bondage or bondage of the entire genital area, for instance, doesn't have any of the feeling of being unable to escape, but it has some very real sensuality all its own. And, in the same way, torture of just the genitals– whether by whipping, electricity, clothespins, stretching, squeezing, weights, or whatever–is a *limited* scene. Some people find that it answers not only their novice trepidations, but their entire hunger for pain scenes.

Along similar lines, while it is not possible to put armpits in bondage per se, it is certainly possible to limit the area of painful torture to the pits. Doing this can lead to a great many discoveries about what is sensually exciting. It can also open pathways to pleasure not likely to be explored by novices who don't set such a limit or make the appropriate request. While there are some important nerves, blood vessels, and tendons in the armpit, they are protected by the depth of their placement in the pit, so pit pain is safe unless super-straining, inward pressure is used. Also, pit-licking is a major pleasure and minor activity in a lot of leathersex scenes. All in all, a fine place to start your SM adventuring.

Nipples are often the first spots the newcomer to leather wants to have manhandled. This is understandable, since just about everyone discovers the possibility of at least mild self-SM through some sort of tit-torture, although they usually don't call it that right away. So, nipples are another area that can be delineated and made the limit for torture or, oddly enough, for bondage. Using "elastrators," veterinary devices intended for castrating barnyard animals, nipples can be raised to beautiful, blood-filled balloons. Using ordinary clothespins, abrasive gloves, fingertips or fingernails, a nail file, piercing needles, and any number of other toys, nipples can become the very center of a bottom's sensual universe for a few hours, or a few days if the torture is intense enough.

Pierced nipples decorated with rings or bars can also be bound by wrapping cord or string around them in such a way that the bindings lift the nipple away from the body. Few things so small can be so pleasantly surprising to look at or toy with as cord-wrapped nipples protruding an inch, eventually more than an inch, out from the chest with nothing but the body jewelry holding the cord in place.

Feet, too, are fine areas for spot torture and limited bondage. In fact, there are a number of national fraternities devoted to helping foot fetishists find and enjoy each other. While feet as fetish are handled in another chapter, playing with feet is not necessarily a fetish activity. Foot bondage and foot torture, like other spot play options, can be both a good way for novices to "test the waters" of leathersex and an interesting permanent play-style.

Spot torture and spot bondage can introduce a touch of leathersex excitement into a night of otherwise vanilla sexual experience. Also, spot torture can be a way of building up or testing a particular partner's essential trustworthiness in the whole realm of pain scenes.

Beyond nipples, genitals, pits, and feet, however, the body can be divided into any number of other spots accessible to torture. This, for some reason, seems to come as a surprise to many men, both novices and experienced players. For example, drumming on the inner thighs for a few seconds may tickle or just be interesting. Drumming away at the same spot, not harder but for a longer time, at least several minutes, can be an ecstatic pain ritual. The most interesting thing in the way of spot torture is to have a regular play partner who will work with you, explore with you, to find the spots on your body that respond with ecstasy rather than agony to prolonged pummelling or other stimulation.

Any number of very pleasurable evenings might be spent in searching out your own personal geography of pleasure. Any body area might turn out to be very erogenous for you: the back of your neck, the sensitive area behind your knees, the arches of your feet, the sacral area at the bottom of your back, the dividing line between your ass cheeks. There is nothing wrong with finding pleasure in any body part, nor is there anything lacking in you if you find no pleasure in the stimulation of body parts other guys say are erotically supercharged.

Obviously, nipples, genitals, pits, and feet top the list of body parts most people like to have attended to by a thoughtful and experienced Top. So long as the man you have in mind is either very experienced or very responsive to your limits, there is no problem involved. And yet, there is a warning due here: If you want to have your cock and balls tortured, be sure your partner knows what he is doing. While nipples can be reduced to hamburger with no real problem (supposing you attend to them as you would any wound) and armpits are relatively safe from genuine damage, the genitals require knowledgeable attention if the scene is going far into the realm of pain.

All of that takes us a little afield from the original idea of spot torture as a limited scene, of course, but rightly so. Many people get into some sort of spot torture because it is small, but adequate to meet their leathersex needs. Then, years later, with lots of experience and many areas of expertise to call on, they are still returning to the spot torture they started with. This is sometimes simply because the pleasures are that inviting. It is also true that alternately limiting and generalizing the area of stimulation can become a bridge to more intense levels of erotic involvement. Let it be what it is for you, so long as a part of what it is can be called pleasure.

BOXING AND BEATING

Wanting to be hurt by being hit is pretty basic physical masochism. Wanting to be hit very hard and repeatedly until you fall over or pass out, on the other hand, is a relatively rare variation on the masochism theme, but it happens. What's more, it is not something that being spanked, caned, whipped, or whacked leads to in any natural progression. In fact, guys who like to be slugged into submission or punched to a knockout are sometimes completely turned off by any other kind of pain trip. They often say they hate the pain, their trip is entirely bound up in the sudden act of being completely conquered. Others continue to enjoy the more common pain scenes, but they don't see heavy beating/KO boxing as the same thing at all.

For some men, all-out punching and slugging is a form of foreplay bound up with something that could be called "fighting for Top" or "loser gets fucked." Usually it is completely inappropriate to think that guys who play this way need the excuse of losing a fight in order to handle the idea of being passive, but there are probably ties to that sort of social conditioning involved.

For other men, heavy beating and boxing are challenges they set themselves, tests of how much they can take, and "take like a man." Again, it may seldom really be appropriate to think of this as seriously playing out the cultural role of the macho male to the limit, but the flavor of that conditioning is certainly present.

Still other guys get into heavy beating and boxing purely because their fantasy images are connected to that sort of thing: to boxers and wrestlers, to "street punk" or cop-criminal types of violent interaction, or to other kinds of out-of-control violence. The important difference being that, in a leathersex/SM setting, the "violence" is ritualized to the point of a certain degree of safety, even if *expressing* the concept of safety is antierotic for these men.

Obviously, beatings that make reference to street fights or professional boxing carry with them the risks and dangers of their real-world counterparts. Being slugged so hard that you pass out, with or without boxing gloves, can easily cause neck and spinal injuries, broken bones, and all sorts of other complications. And still, I know of at least two men who come in the split second before they pass out, when they feel the right punch connect. One of them claims that he never comes any other way.

Even if they both experience orgasms as they pass out, my knockout pals are not that much alike in another important aspect of their heavy beating scenes. One wants to be restrained either with enforced orders or chains so he won't have the opportunity to hit back. The other absolutely requires that he be free to strike back, although he will pull his own punches as much as necessary to be sure that he gets the punch he wants without hurting the man who is offering to give it to him. Another option here, mentioned above, is that some guys want the outcome of the fight to be uncertain, or at least to seem so.

When we're talking about action that carries as much risk of injury and as many opportunities for loss of control as is the case with beating/boxing, we're sure to run into a lot of men who will say that it isn't properly SM. They'll tell us anything that dangerous has to be considered beyond the realm of action that can be safe enough and sane enough to ever be truly consensual. But these guys are basically laying on their leathersex soul mates the same argument the vanilla world gives all of us: If it isn't interesting and sexual and enjoyable for me, it isn't good, it isn't sex, and it shouldn't be done.

No matter what gets your dick hard, so long as you can find sane partners who genuinely want to do it with you, and so long as you are able to reduce the risks to a level you and your partners are willing to accept, you can't let yourself become too attentive to the outsiders' arguments against it. If wrestling and boxing are acceptable as athletic events (or entertainments), it must be possible to do the same things at home—with or without erotic intentions—and it is.

It is almost never productive to get involved with asking why people do the leathersex things they do. After all, if they keep doing something, it has to be because they like it and want more of it, and that alone is answer enough. But some kinds of leathersex have bonuses that are completely understandable.

Pain scenes, in particular, engage the still-mysterious, naturally occurring opiates that are part of our bodies' pain management systems. These internally produced drugs can be very pleasant. They are, no doubt, part of what is at work in a lot of spiritual disciplines involving intense physical activities and pains. And, until the last mysteries of the human soul are explained away, there will be people who will do whatever it takes to get these substances pumped into their blood and brain. What it comes down to, over and over, is that we do what gets us high, what gets us off, and what leaves us feeling good. For some people, the high is only (or most directly) accessible when the action is very heavy or very scary. So be it.

ELECTRICITY

Electricity is everywhere, no problem. Then, someone suggests SM play with electricity. Suddenly, visions of the electric chair appear in our brains, along with thoughts of people being struck by lightning, doctors zapping heart patients with electric paddles, all those warnings against sticking your tongue into an outlet when you were learning to crawl, and the scary labels on ordinary appliances: "Danger! Warn children of the risk of death by electric shock."

Yeah, electricity is mysterious stuff, all right, and never more strange and wonderful than when it is coursing through the cock and balls of a well-endowed man who is neatly tied down and handsomely struggling against the bondage.

Actually, electricity is one of the safer ways to play, the jitters from all those warnings being, for the novice, a part of the scene, apparently.

There are three ways to play with electricity. The simplest is just to use toys that happen to be electrical: vibrating dildoes, jiggling tit clamps, heating pads, and the like. Since electricity doesn't directly contact the body, these are not, in a strict sense, playing with electricity itself.

The second kind of electrical play involves only static electricity. Violet Wands are the most common static toys on the market and surely the most fun for relatively easy, low-level electrical play with nearly complete safety. Static, after all, is only static. There is no current going anywhere in the body, so it cannot go to the wrong internal organs or screw up your biological circuitry. It is entirely superficial stimulation so, although you can get a burn by playing at top intensity in a single spot for a long time, you aren't going to cause any internal injury or *any* damage that is not immediately obvious, and avoidable.

Violet Wands have been around for about 100 years. They are "health and beauty" appliances, originally sold to cure everything from baldness and rashes to cataracts and tooth decay. No one ever proved there were any actual health benefits from Violet Wands–not along the lines promised by the creators of the device, anyway–but someone has continued to buy wands in sufficient quantities to keep the product available for a century. (Hmmm. Now, who could possibly be buying these things? Heh-heh.)

The other way to play with electricity is actual currents of AC (US house current) or DC (batteries) power, applied directly to the body. There is, obviously, a lot of highly technical information that one might enjoy having on the subject of electricity, but–just as you don't need to know the inner workings of a computer to type and print a letter–you don't need to know how electricity works in any detail to play safely. There is no need to experiment with rewired toasters, or anything of the sort. Very good, made-for-SM toys are easily available.

What you need for electrical play is a power source, one or more sets of connecting cables, and some attachments to make the appropriate contacts with the desired body parts.

The power source will be either a battery-powered control box, or a plug-in unit with a step-down converter and controls. Such units are available from leather stores and SM supply houses. Once you know what you're doing you may want to play with Relax-a-cisors and other "health and beauty" appliances that provide pulsing current, but start with a box made to supply power for leathersex play. The cables are usually pairs of light wires with plugs appropriate to the power box on one end and clips, plugs, or bare wire on the other end, depending how and with what attachments you intend to play. The attachments can be anything from copper pipes and chromed clothespins, to metal dildoes, alligator clips, and specially created items like electrifiable cockrings, urethral inserts, and butt plugs. The best attachments are made for the very kind of play you want, and they're sold by SM supply houses, often by mail.

To play, you simply attach the ends of two leads (cables) from the same control box circuit to two body points, using a water-based gel to improve electrical conductivity. For example, you slip into a made-for-electro-play cockring, and pop a similar butt plug into your ass; attach the leads to these; and start experimenting with the controls–which you kept set at their lowest level until you turned on the power. Good control boxes let you vary both the level of the electricity and the rate at which it pulses. Your choices run from barely perceptible, buzzy stimulation to muscle-wracking jolts of painful torture.

One warning, and if you are using SM-specific electrical toys no other is required: don't let the circuitry get set up in such a way that you are passing current through the chest cavity where it may interfere with your heart's naturally rhythmic electric pulses. Even this warning may prove unnecessary when you have appropriate training from an experienced player.

That's it. Go play now. You can play with yourself, very nicely, with electricity. You can experiment on yourself as a way of preparing to play with someone else. Or you can let someone else (who has presumably already done some experimenting) play with you. That's the ticket, let someone else do the work.

CIGARS AND CIGARETTES

Cigar fetishes are getting remarkably popular. The reason may have a great deal to do with the aging of the baby boomers, the "American Dream" image of Dad in the decades when today's leathersex perverts were growing up, or it may have nothing to do with anything so distinct. Cigarettes in leathersex scenes, at the same time, are all but disappearing. This, almost certainly, has a lot to do with the currently raging social stigma on smokers, and the embarrassment cigarette smokers are expected (rightly or not) to feel when they light up.

Fetishes, while they are not the subject of this chapter, sometimes play a significant role in setting up the power exchange for the pain scenes that are done with cigars, cigarettes, and lighters. Some of these scenes depend on the masculine image–Dad with his smokes–that the bottom carries with him. Others, no less significantly, have to do with the Top's version of smoking as an identifier of the "man in charge," or with his possibly unconscious image of himself as a fearless, fire-handling man–a sort of modern Prometheus. Finally, for both Tops and bottoms, smoking can become erotically charged just because it is so distant from their everyday lives. So, some nonsmoking Tops light up in the dungeon to fulfill the bottom's image of Dad or their own, or to create a Promethean self-image, or to powerfully distinguish themselves *as SM players* from themselves as accountants or store clerks.

Fetish involvement aside, the pain scenes associated with cigarettes are usually more extreme than those associated with cigars. A cigar can be waved around like a magic wand, trailing the threat of serious burns and a constant, blunt knifelike pain wherever it goes. Of course, like cigarettes, cigars can be put out against skin, but the burns from this *can be* so severe that most guys find ways to play with cigars that don't involve pressing and holding the burning end of the cigar against the bottom's skin. Cigarettes don't work nearly so well as heat wands or threats–except with easily scared bottoms–so they are often pushed to the extreme of being crushed out on the skin as a way of getting some sensation value out of them.

Of course, for the sake of confirming domination, asserting power, or imposing humiliation, a Top might also make his boy eat the butts of his cigars or cigarettes, or take flipped off ashes on his tongue. The former is questionable. Certainly tobacco butts are not health food. The latter is a nearly harmless delight. "Boy, tongue!" The tongue is instantly presented, of course. While the boy may expect a boot, a cock head, an asshole, or whatever, what he gets is spent ash dropped on his tongue. The warmth can shock as though it burned–and if the Top flips too hard, he can obviously knock loose burning tobacco and cause serious burning!–but, usually, the warmth is almost immediately blotted out by the repugnant taste and texture of the clean, dissolving ash.

As with any scene incorporating heat, it is very advisable to have either very slowly and carefully developed experience, or carefully presented training for cigar and cigarette scenes. The possibility of doing unintended damage is always there, as is the possibility of producing shock states that are out of all proportion to the visible action.

To play with an open flame such as a lighter rather than the lit end of a cigar or cigarette is to play with the same scene raised to the tenth power, at least. While all risks are yours to judge and sort out for yourself, you have to take all warnings about playing with fire very seriously. The burns are to be expected, but they can be surprisingly severe, and you have to be ready to deal with burns that are much more severe than you expected. More surprising still–especially if flames come into a scene after a good deal of other psychologically disorienting play–is the way that even the smallest flame can set off primal screams and primitive fears. These reactive states are next to impossible to be prepared for, but you have to be ready for anything if you must play with fire.

Speaking of preparedness, it is irresponsible to play with any fire-hot heat, including a lit cigarette, unless you have a fire extinguisher in the room. You can't guess all the things that may happen, and many of the possible eventualities can result in your heat source–cigar, cigarette, or lighter– transferring a flame-producing energy to something else.

Until now we haven't talked much of political correctness, but the relationship is very rare in which a bottom will accept a Top's right to do something which he has been told *on the evening news* is unsafe. Secondhand smoke is famously unsafe, so be prepared for the leathersex partner who will say that you may castrate him with rusty pruning shears if you like, but you may not smoke in the play space. After all, surgery with rusty shears has not been much mentioned by the major network news programs.

PIERCING

When you meet a man with piercing eyes, you're nailed. You feel he can see right through you, and you might very well like that. When you meet a man with piercing on his mind, you're in for quite a ride. If you get together to have a go at it, he'll be pushing pins and needles right through you, and you'd better have a pretty good idea in advance of whether he knows what he's doing, *and* whether you really want to explore the area of having things stuck into or through your skin, muscles, and protruding parts.

Piercing has come a long way in the past decade or two. Once upon a time, not so long ago, any piercing except pairs of female earlobes was something we associated with tribal kingdoms far, far away either in time or geography. Now, the tribe of leatherfolk in Everytown, USA, is sporting gold and silver rings here, there, and everywhere.

If you can pinch it, they say, pierce it, and they do . . . we do. Although that modern saying is sometimes pronounced rather glibly, it is true enough. A play piercing might sometimes be done in an area that cannot be pinched up between the thumb and a finger tip comfortably, but piercings that are meant to stay in need to be in areas where they are not resisted by the tension of the tissue trying to return to its pre-pierced contours. So, if you can pinch it, pierce it, works *up to a point*. Even so, if you have to work at getting a hold of a body part to pinch it, you'll probably see any piercing there ease itself to the surface and grow out in time, although it may still be a good place for play piercings that are removed at the end of the scene.

Ears aside, pierced nipples predominate, it seems, with Prince Albert piercings (in through the urethra, out through the underside of the cock) holding a close second among guys I know. And there are more piercings in more body parts showing up all the time. This is fine, of course, but no matter how common body piercing has become, it has *not* become easier or safer in any way. Expert training is still needed before anyone should attempt permanent piercings, meaning ones in which jewelry will be worn. And, even for temporary or play piercings, a great deal of technical information is required to keep the procedures safe.

Fortunately, training is not all that hard to come by. It can be arranged in the form of lessons from any number of experienced piercers all over the country. It can also be acquired in the process of having oneself turned into a walking erotic jewelry display, by any number of experienced piercers. Failing live training, Master Piercer Jim Ward (Gauntlet Inc. of Los Angeles, San Francisco, and New York) has made some excellent instructional videos. So, now that we know you are *not* going to go out and start poking needles in anyone–even yourself–without special preparation, we can concentrate on you being the piercer's subject. The pierc*ee?*

Getting into a play piercing scene per se is not necessarily the way to sample the joys of the form, especially since many play-piercing Tops want to do dozens, even hundreds of temporary piercings in a single scene. But you might be able to negotiate a taste of piercing–play piercing–in a scene that has many elements. That way, if the needles don't do it for you, you still have the likelihood of a satisfying scene.

Finding a competent, fully prepared play-piercing Top may not be easy, but permanent piercings, on the other hand, are . . . well, they're permanent. This means, if nothing else, that you ought to think about why you want to be pierced before you jump into it.

The possibilities are endless, but experiencing the pain is one of the poorer reasons for undertaking a permanent piercing. Sometimes, the scene of a permanent piercing can be turned into a ceremony, a ritual of laying claim to one's own body, or of installing jewelry to mark a special personal passage or to memorialize a special person or event. Sometimes people are pierced just because they like the look of nipple rings or a Prince Albert, or because they enjoy the shock value of a pierced eyebrow, nose, or interfinger web. Not infrequently, a bottom is pierced to please his Top, Master, owner, or keeper. And it isn't unheard of for a guy to get his first piercings because he has heard about the effect it has on "the internal wiring," the way that, after a piercing, some guys experience a sudden and seemingly permanent jump in their erotic sensibilities, or a reinvigoration of their sexual interest, or a new outlook on the connection between their bodies and their spiritual aspirations.

Think along these lines, and give fair time to whatever other thoughts come to mind, as you consider why you might want to be pierced. Then, whatever the reason, do it for that considered and determined reason.

The next consideration is where, by whom, and under what circumstances you want a piercing. Often your reason for wanting the piercing will help with this series of choices. If you're being pierced *for* your Master, of course, you probably won't be involved in these decisions. But, if the choices are yours, consider this. Ritualizing a piercing is best done elsewhere than in a jewelry store, but getting an expert piercing quickly and easily is best done in a store or piercer's workspace.

One of the options that is always available is that you may want your permanent piercing to be part of a leathersex scene. There is nothing particularly wrong with this so long as the piercer is knowledgeable about appropriate cautions and hygiene, which may very well mean that the piercer and the play partner are not the same person. It is not unusual for a person to make this arrangement, in fact: Top A and bottom b invite piercer C to their scene, to participate only in the piercing. Things proceed as ritually or casually as intended until, at some point, the piercing is accomplished. Then A and B go on about their erotic business, while C cleans up and clears out.

Remember, one Master of anything is worth 100 or more people who attempt it. So, you are not a piercer until a Master Piercer tells you that you are, or until, after careful study of whatever sort, 100 bottoms you have pierced unanimously agree that you know what you are doing. But, you can master the art of enjoying piercing–being pierced, that is–rather handily, just by checking it out, finding it fun, and deciding to submit to a reliable, piercing-fanatic Top.

Here's the scene: You say yes, he gets a pin cushion for the night–you. The other stuff you want to negotiate for this kind of scene is easy. Will you be tied up while he works? Say "yes," it's more fun that way, and it's always easier to go on for a while with a fun scene than a boring one. Will he be providing other stimulation (what stone-cold outsiders call pain) during the scene? Say "yes,"

again, specifying the type of stimulation you want, usually by letting him suggest things until you accept something. (After all, the
power exchange works better if you let the Top have the feeling that
everything is his idea, and that he's getting his way, exactly.) And,
will he be attaching weights, stretching cords, or otherwise *using*
the temporary piercings once they are in place? Try to say yes to
this one too, but this is an area worthy of discussion before you go
any further.

You may find that you have some limits about how many piercings you can deal with. In point of fact, if the piercing is done
expertly (and it *must* be), your limit is going to be more psychological than physical. That is, if the idea of being pierced gets you high,
there's no reason why there should be much difference between one
play piercing and 50 or more, if the pace and atmosphere are carefully managed. Be sure you have some way of signaling that you
need him to slow down or work on another body area for a while,
something like a specially devised safe word will do, or just permission–within the nature of the scene, as always–to speak frankly
about this.

You may also find that you have definite limits as to how much
the play piercings can be handled, tugged at, weighted down,
wrapped with cords, or otherwise "tortured." This is going to be
mostly a physical question–your pain/stimulation limits. Here's
how to cope with the scene becoming intense, which is good, without having it push you over your limits, rather than expanding them:
Using the safe word mentioned above, take responsibility for managing your own stimulation level and the pace at which it increases,
unless your Top is brilliant in this area, and *honestly* doesn't need
your help. If you go at it slowly enough, both in terms of the overall
pace and the movement between body parts, you can get to the
endorphin high (pain-suppressing rush) by the time the piercings
are all in place. This, by the way, is a good reason to choose to let
the Top do lots of piercings rather than just a few.

Once you're into the high that eases over you from comfortably
allowing the stimulation (stabbing) to continue long enough and
intensely enough, accept as much stroking, touching, and slight
manipulation of the piercings as you can. This will confirm and
intensify your rush and your comfort. It will also help the Top to

pace the action, as he will get a lot of physical feedback from this phase of the scene.

Now, you're high but still effectively experiencing the scene, and he's getting off on his handiwork (why else would he bother?). If he wants to interlace the piercings to create a trussed bondage, to give himself a harp-like instrument to play, or just to watch you wiggle as he does it, you'll be able to handle it, or to know with certainty that you can't handle it. Through it all, even when you are thinking it has already been enough, pacing is everything. This is a scene where your "no" might mean "give me a few minutes to get ready for it."

Ready to put the scene into hyper-drive? The Top can pull back some of the needles that have already been inserted, allowing their tips to be left under the skin this time. Now, in addition to the stimulation of the piercing and the added sensations already mentioned, piercing becomes a genuine pain trip, and a fairly extreme one, too.

If the needles are manipulated with their tips under the skin rather than poking out half an inch or so from where they were inserted, the slightest movement is exquisitely painful. This is a very elegant, highly controllable pain trip, using tiny areas inside the body in addition to the insertion site. And each needle is an area that can be separately stimulated. (Note: The tips of the needles may need to be chemically resterilized before they are pulled back under the skin, whether to be left there for a while or for removal.)

Thrilling just to think about being a pin cushion like this, no? Yes! And, the only real safety warning required is that you know your Top knows what he is doing physically and in terms of sterile conditions. After the scene, depending on your predictable rate of healing, you may need to keep the piercing sites especially clean, or even medicate them, but that just stretches the sensations of the scene over the next several days. Good!

BINDING AND CORSETING

When bondage becomes painful, it is usually a sign of trouble. A restraint may need to be repositioned, a rope loosened, or some postural demand of the bondage may need to be relieved. In some leathersex situations, however, bindings are intended to cause pain or discomfort, and this always increases the demand for stamina in the bottom and expertise in the Top. The major overlapping categories of play in which bindings are used to create sensation, rather than merely to restrain the bottom, can be called painful bondage, tight bindings, and corseting.

Painful bondage is not just regular bondage gone awry and left that way. That would just be called *bad* bondage. An overly tight wrist restraint, for instance, causes pain only when there is a real risk of damage. Instead, painful bondage is any system of ropes or other restraints that is intended both to limit the bottom's freedom of movement *and* produce sensations–understood as controlled pain. Only the most vigilant and expert Top can create a bondage that is able to restrain, cause pain, *and* be used to keep the bottom available for some other sort of leathersex attention like a flogging. The jolting of a flogging would be changing the conditions of the bondage, reducing the Top's actual control of the situation, and perhaps leaving the bottom confused as to what is intended and what both he and his Top might be regretting later.

In painful bondage, the pain is not the result of pressure on joints or bones. It might come from strategically placed knots in ropes that pass tightly over large muscles, or from thinner cords running between restraints, crossing and compressing muscle masses. But whatever it is, painful bondage produces the desired pain in the same safe-to-torture body parts as any other pain scene. In its most elegant application, painful bondage is only slightly discomforting (if at all) when it is installed. The pain develops over time, as it does when you must sit too long in an uncomfortable theatre seat. A brilliant Top can develop a scene in which he is ready to let up on some other ministrations at about the time he can predict the effects of the painful bondage are adequate to "take over for him." Less brilliant Tops can use the same idea, carefully reading the bottom's responses, and getting out of the way of the bondage pain as it comes on. The finesse called for is extreme, but worth learning. Besides, in this case, there is no other way to learn but by doing.

Tight bindings are different from bondage primarily in that they are not used to tie the bottom to anything–even himself–for the purpose of restricting movement. These bindings are their own excuse for being. Such bindings, at their best, are done with thin ropes or even package twine, looped over the major muscles in a carefully designed, repeating pattern. They interfere with surface blood circulation, but don't starve the tissues of essential blood supplies. They cause surface marking and irritation, but don't break the skin. They cause discomforts that can be prolonged for hours, but they don't cause any damage. Obviously, to do this requires special training. If the only available teacher is experience, that experience must be carefully controlled, building slowly on observations and postscene discussions.

Corseting is a still more specialized form of painful binding. As it is used here, the term refers not only to corsets themselves, but to bindings which are, relative to the body part involved, broad enough that they produce even squeezing rather than the "cutting" effect of a thin cord. The waist line is not the only possible area for corseting.

While bondage of any sort can be either the scene itself or a way to facilitate or intensify some other scene, most painful bindings are used only when the bottom is able to remain stationary or nearly so. Corseting can often be a *mobile* pain trip. If an actual corset or materials approximating a corset are used around the waist, for example, the constricted bottom can then be taken out to the bar wearing loose clothing. No one knows that he is conscious of every breath he takes, and constantly adjusting his posture to control pain, but you and he know that you are in charge of him at a very intimate level, even when you walk away and leave him chatting with friends.

Corseting, of course, is not a novice-Top trip. It requires tremendous sensitivity and self-restraint, as well as a solid grasp of the limiting physiological factors. Corset-like wraps on feet, hands, thighs, upper arms, etc., are frequently done with elastic bandages or strips of latex. These, too, demand a great deal from the responsible party—meaning the Top when two or more are playing. If you put such wrappings on yourself—and you probably shouldn't—be sure that you do so in such a way that you will be able to release them quickly, wherever you are, in the event that a panic state comes over you, or for any other reason.

When playing with binding and corseting, there are many ways you might end up interfering unintentionally with the body's normal and necessary functions. Besides relatively benign constriction of surface blood flow, even carefully placed corsets can unduly push on internal organs and disarrange or dangerously stress bones. That places this kind of play on the short list of leathersex games which really ought to be undertaken only by experts, under expert guidance, or by the most sensitive and observant players.

USING OR PROCESSING PAIN

Pain is mysterious stuff, and everyone reacts differently to it. If five guys get more or less the same thump on the heel from the same overwound automatic door closer, one will glance behind himself and go on to his next appointment; another will wince, shrug, and limp a bit; another will need pain relief medication; another will take the day off from the office; and another will sue for millions (or threaten to do so), limping and complaining and even actually aching for days. If the same five guys see someone else in pain, (no, it's not another countdown!), their reactions might range from smothering sympathy to the genuine belief that the only way to get over the pain is to ignore it and get on with what you were doing.

What is intolerable pain to one person is a cozily welcome midnight reminder of a hard-played afternoon football game to another. And yet, presented with the idea that there are people who seek pain, who get high on pain, and who get hard from pain, even the look-a'-my-bruises football player will usually react with disgust. In fact, if athletes could think of SM as sports, they'd understand the acceptance of pain, but they'd always want to know who was winning. If executives who are willing to stare at columns of tiny numerals till their heads are about to burst and their eyes are watering could think of SM as business, they'd understand the acceptance of pain, but they'd always want to know who was profiting from whom.

SM, though, is neither a sport nor a business (not as such, not usually), so it mystifies and disgusts. Not that they're more likely to understand, but it might be better to take the question of pain to a gardener rather than to athletes and businessmen. He or she would understand the idea, if not the actuality quickly enough: Pain is the weed-word of sensation. Last year's carnations are unwanted when they push up among this year's tidy rows of pansies. They are weeds. They are plants not wanted in this place at this time. Just so, pain can be seen as a sensation that is not welcome at a particular time, coming in the way it does. But, just as the carnations are still flowers, pain is still a sensation; and, just as a gardener might choose to accommodate or move the pesky carnations, a masochist is able to process and use sensations that others would dismiss as pain.

So, the eternal question arises, the one that has to be asked at just about every SM demonstration-lecture: If a masochist gets hit by a car, does he enjoy it? No. It's as simple as that. No, a masochist does not enjoy being injured accidentally. His experience with pain may make him better able than most people to understand how badly injured he is, to know what kind of care he is likely to need, and even to bear the pain. None of which should suggest that an SM bottom wants, seeks, enjoys, or puts up with accidental injury any more than anyone else. That sort of sensory experience is a weed. It is pain.

SM bottoms learn very quickly what kinds of stimulation and sensation they do and don't want. They learn almost as quickly how to encourage Tops to give them the stimulation they want and to prevent Tops from providing sensations they want to avoid. (The grey areas between what a guy wants and what he wants to avoid are negotiable, more often than not.) What bottoms learn less quickly is how to process the intense sensation–okay, *pain*–so that they can bear more of it for a longer time, get more of the pleasure that makes pain-seeking attractive, and have a better shot at some of the better Tops (who will very likely want a guy who can take enough of a scene to get them off, too).

Processing pain, at least to a certain extent, is natural. If it were not, even a hangnail could bring the toughest bruiser to his knees (come on guys, you wouldn't want that for *yourself* so don't go wishing it on the big boys). For some people–boys more than girls–an additional degree of pain processing is taught from a very early age, but not always in the healthiest way. Then there are the lucky few who, once they become involved in SM, intentionally continue their education in pain processing by noticing what works, and developing that; noticing what others do, and trying that; and by asking questions or taking classes to increase their pain-handling capabilities.

How a person goes about processing intense sensation into a tide of pleasure depends on what kind of person he is to begin with. Some people respond to pain with nothing short of "Oh, boy!" These are true masochists; processing pain is not an issue. What they need is to be told how to get more of the specific type of pain they want. Others react with "Oh, yeah?" These guys are going to fight for the Top position (even if it is an obviously foregone conclusion who will win the fight, and it isn't always). If they lose (was there ever any doubt?), these guys are going to "take it like men," which is a very rudimentary and fairly ineffective way of processing pain. In fact, a lot of men learn to give the impression that they are toughing it out like good little soldiers when, actually, they have learned and are using much more sophisticated pain processing methods.

Another initial reaction to pain in the playroom is "Oh, no!" This comes from people who, supposing they knew what they were getting into, need help. They need to learn by heart the path from whack to heaven, and it will be hard if they can't shed their oh-no attitude. And, finally, there are people who react to the prospect of pain with nothing heartier than "Oh, well." Chances are they will never be bothered to learn how to handle, use, and enjoy the ministrations of a good Top. Until they stop soaking up the hot SM energy and go back to the excitement of word-search puzzles, they will be yawning while one Top after another wears himself out at the other end of a whip or whatever.

HOW PAIN IS HANDLED

Strangely, the ways people process pain are often considered more personal than the most graphic details of their sex lives. Maybe the highly guarded privacy gathers around pain handling because processing pain seems to imply that the bottom "needs help" which he ought to be glad to manage without. Or, maybe the problem is simply that, because we don't often speak of it, we haven't developed a comfortable language in which to tell each other about our pain-processing successes and failures, methods and magic. Whatever the reason, most people prefer not to talk about the pain processing techniques they use or the unconscious processes they observe in themselves. Nonetheless, it is not difficult to describe a few ways to juggle pain while spinning it into pleasure.

Breath

With TV motherhood in graphic and perennial bloom, you don't need ever to have known a pregnant woman to know that they are told to "breathe, breathe, breathe" in order to cope with the pains of labor and giving birth. Why they should have to be told is another question since every little kid in the world seems to instinctively understand that huffing, puffing, and sucking deep breaths changes the way a smashed fingertip feels. Not surprisingly, breath is the most common vehicle for pain control in SM play, too.

Generally, the idea is to breathe out the pain, and breathe in a relaxed receptivity to the scene in progress. There is no point in asking whether this, or any pain processing method for that matter, is more imagination or medicine, visualization or self-delusion. The point is that it works. Engaging the palpable sense of bodily presence initiated by the introduction of the painful stimulation, the process is simple: locate the breath within the body as a gatherer of the pain, deliver it to the lungs, and release pain and spent air together.

If for no other reason, this method is bound to be effective with early stages and low levels of pain just because it stands as a reminder to breathe and to breathe deeply. When we breathe deeply, we are doing a more effective job of heat exchanging between the surrounding environment and the interior of our bodies, and mild trauma is often greeted with a slightly elevated body temperature. Not that anything is explained away by that fact, but it may help the skeptic engage his imagination and put breath to work in SM.

Fantasy

Some people find that pain is managed when they submerge themselves in the right fantasy role. A person being flogged, for example, casts himself in the role of the Roman galley slave for whom the pain of a flogging (history be damned) is an everyday experience. Since it is nothing out of the ordinary, it is nothing all that disquieting. In the end, it is tolerated. Whether this path to *bearing* pain closes some of the doors to pleasure is very debatable. Some guys claim that they don't notice when the role ceases to be used, or necessary. For them, then, role playing (even if no one else knows they are doing it) serves a purpose, very likely either keeping them occupied until the body begins to handle the pain in its own way, or acting as a cover for unconscious pain-processing methods they may not appreciate.

Heat, Light, and Color

Heat is naturally generated in the body by most methods of stimulation. Whether it is slapped with a paddle, scoured with an abrasive toy, pinched, stretched, or punctured, the body sends its investigative reporters (armies of blood cells) to the sight of the trauma, and blood is the heat-carrier. So, it is not much of a leap to identify pain with heat. Just about everybody can do it, and that is the beginning of a rather simple method of pain processing.

To experience heat as light is also a relatively easy step. Even speaking scientifically the distinction between what we ordinarily experience as heat and what we call light is a matter of perception as much as anything. Similarly, to assign a color designation to any experience of heat or light is well within the realm of normal imaginative capabilities. So, pain processing methods that work with heat can also be performed with light and color.

There are three distinct options available here, and combinations of two or three of them are not uncommon either. First, heat (which will stand for color and light as well at the moment) can be generalized. Just as a towel is less "wet" when the water in it has spread by capillary action over a large area of its fibers, pain is less intense when it is experienced over a larger area of the body. Some people find it very easy to recognize the pain of a single blow in a specific area, then to release that pain so it can spread over a larger area, perhaps even being driven over still larger areas with each successive blow. A good Top, recognizing that a bottom is having trouble dealing with the immediate pain will often stroke the reddened skin outward from the center, not to soothe per se so much as to encourage the generalizing of the pain over a larger area. For this tech-

nique to work, the bottom needs nothing more than the intention
that it should, and a modicum of imagination.

Next, the heat (light, color) can be drawn to the surface. This
operation may require more imagination, and it seems to have less
science in it than most, but it works for some people. Here the
experience of pain as heat, for example, is pressed outward from
within the body, leaving the heat on the surface. Superficial pain is,
almost by definition, tolerable. That is the primary force behind the
effectiveness of this method, and a certain amount of its appeal
comes from the fact that we have seen superficial injuries heal all
our lives, but we retain (and should!) a fear of internal injury. In
fact, if a pain is only skin deep, how could anyone possibly find it
intolerable, especially if managing that pain means that the scene
goes on (with a man who happens to be hot enough to have gotten
the scene going in the first place)?

Heat, light, and–as a kind of light–color, can also be radiated. In
fact, they actually are radiated from the body in their various ways
all the time. Where generalizing spread the transformed pain around
the body, and superficializing brought it out like a shell encasing the
body, radiating expels the pain. There is, of course, a still higher
degree of imaginative capacity called for here, but it is not beyond
the sort of imagination required for most formal meditations.
Whether it is sensed as heat, light, or a defined color, the pain can be
radiated outward from the source–however superficial or deep
within the body. This not only reduces the experience of the pain as
pain, but it tends to encourage the experience of joy in the leathersex scene, and to connect leathersex with the most effortless kind of
letting go, which multiplies the opportunities for SM joy.

Storage

A lot of people, especially novices, have trouble identifying pain
with anything as welcome as heat, light, or color; they can't deal
with fantasy roles, or let go enough to use them; and they find their
breath more often pushing them toward weed-pain than lifting them
away from it. And yet, they are getting something they "know"
they want. They wonder if they really want it, but keep coming back
in search of more of what is more or less the same thing. Sadly, they

also often blame their Tops for not teaching them how to cope, or for not "doing it so it feels good."

For these people, one method of pain processing that is almost always accessible is this: store the energy of the pain in or near the site where it is being originated, and let it build up without resisting it. Give your attention to retaining full awareness of the sensation and of the fact that it is exactly what you bargained for, holding on to it as long as possible. Then, having warned your Top of this moment before the scene began, you can signal (perhaps with a safe word) that it is time to release the stored up energy. Release it by shuddering if that comes naturally, shaking if you need to, screaming, squealing, wriggling, or whatever it takes, but remain aware that this is not meant to be a mad scene, just a complete release of stored energy.

Minor variations on this technique are obvious. Bottoms who scream and squeal, wriggle and shudder all through a scene without any encouragement are evidently performing energy releases all the time. This may be distressing for the Top. It may be distracting for other players in the room. It may even be destructive of the entire leathersex atmosphere. Or not. It depends on the nature of the release activity, the intensity of it, and the attitude of the Top and others present. But the bad thing is that it is probably stealing all the more intense experiences from the bottom. Releasing your pain-delivered energy, stroke by stroke as it is received, is like spending your money dollar by dollar as it is earned: You never get to use it to buy anything big enough to wish for.

There are endless possible combinations of these pain processing techniques, and countless other methods as well, but the idea is to process the sensation intentionally, engaging your attention. When you do that, you collect a kind of sensual dividend on the processed energy. The very act of attending to (or even attempting) the processing of sensation has soothing effects on the mind and quiets fearful voices in the head. It encourages good habits of breathing and centered presence, drawing you into the scene, opening you to its possibilities rather than letting you stew on its unlikely side effects.

Perhaps the most significant aspect of pain processing, apart from its involvement in the spiritual aspect of leathersex (discussed in Chapter Eight), is that it gives the bottom the freedom to become a fully contributing partner in the scene. A guy whose only concern is bearing the pain, or when and how to stop it, is not cooperating. He's just wearing down a Top. The same guy in the same scene, when he's engaged in handling the sensations for himself, gets a clearer picture of what is being done to and for him. He has more consciousness free to communicate with the Top, instead of relying on the Top to read his mind (although good Tops do seem to be able to do this). He has liberty where he imagined limits, permitting a longer, more intense, and more satisfying scene for both parties.

Chapter Four

Playing with Pleasure

Somehow it is easier for most people to think of leathermen whipping each other than doing anything that could be called playing with pleasure. Pain scenes though, however important, are not the only options for leathersex. There arc lots of other ways to play. Activities associated with fetishes, for instance, can engage and maintain a significant exchange of power between two men without tending in the least toward pain.

FETISHES IN THE FLESH

What do you look at when you're looking at a man who turns you on? Eyes? Most people say they look at the eyes. The bulge in the front of his pants? Most people seem to think that's where everyone else looks first. Or maybe you look for muscles, height, fur or some other detail of anatomy or costume that starts your juices flowing. Whatever it is, of course, you're not going to change that little kink in your make-up just because you might add leathersex to your repertoire. You may even find that leathermen are more receptive than others to entertaining your special interest, even helping you develop it beyond your wildest dream. Becoming too hung up on a single feature or body part can be limiting, but getting the most from your fetish can only improve your sex life.

For a man with a leathersexual attitude, everybody has good parts, and some parts are almost universally good. An armpit, for example, is either as clean or as smelly as you like an armpit to be, as smoothly shaved, bristly, or hairy as you want. It can be a perfect armpit, even if the man who sports it is not your idea of Adonis. If what you want is to bury your face in one pit after another, then it is probably more important that the man you are with likes your pit licking than that he have a classically handsome face.

Feet, too. A man's feet may be spectacular, even if he has a concave chest, a bird-perch nose, and 23 other "defects" you wouldn't otherwise overlook. Lots of people who may have been uncomfortable with their own foot fetishes before, have discovered that while they were nervous about oral-genital sex for health reasons, eating feet became a passion. Then, condoms and health news aside, they stuck with feet for at least part of their oral play. Including feet in your oral repertoire is easy and fun, especially if you are already into boot service (or fantasize about that) or if you have discovered the pleasures of having a few fingers or a whole hand reaching for your tonsils.

Bootlicking as a demonstration of submission is a normal element of leathersex encounters, but it doesn't always mean that either party has a special interest in feet or boots, nor does a special interest necessarily amount to a fetish. Nonetheless, feet and footgear are such common fetishes that there are local and national organizations with thousands of members who share this special taste. Different foot-men have different interests. Some are satisfied with ordinary bootlicking and the care their Tops demand for their boots. Others want bare feet in their mouths, or kicking them, walking on them, even the feet rather than hands over their mouths and noses in a breath-control scene. Others have the same range of wishes involving feet in particular kinds of socks, in tennis shoes, wingtips, athletic shoes or whatever.

The idea of playing with a man's body one part at a time is simple. You show him how interested you are in the body parts you want to touch, kiss, worship, or abuse, and you do everything in your power to create a pleasurable reaction in him by the attention you give that body part. If you're broad-minded (meaning, not too terribly hung up on the *one* body part) you can give a man the experience of a lifetime by moving from his feet to, say, his nipples, his pits, his fingers, his balls, maybe, then his neck, his hair, (giving special attention to the body part of your special interest) . . . and, eventually, down and around, to the usual focus points of sexual pleasure.

What it's about is finding what turns you on–say, feet–and play-ing at that in such a way that you will be invited to do so again. For the guy whose feet or pits or nipples are the object of your attention, the possibilities are obvious. He can return the favor, at the same time or at a later time; he can remain impassive, leaving you to your own devices; or, if he has the right kind of enthusiasm, he can turn your service to his body part(s) into a full-fledged, power-exchang-ing leathersex scene.

This is very safe sex in almost any form or context. Most skin disorders cause no orally introducible internal disease. If they did little kids who are always licking and chewing at their wounds, sores and rashes would never grow up to be happy perverts (and some of us did). As for HIV infection, the medical community swept away the fear of sweat long ago. Nonetheless, you may very well like to avoid any rough play with eruptions or sores on the skin both to avoid hampering the healing process in your partner and to reduce to nothing any minor risks to yourself.

To the extent that we are really talking about health here, the greater risk to your well-being is this: to have a passionate interest and keep it bottled up. So don't. You may have licked boots, wish-ing all the time for the warm skin beneath. You may have caught a whiff of a date's manly musk and flashed on the desire to bury your face at its sweaty source. You may have watched accumulated moisture trickle down *his* chest and belly to disappear into the waistband of his jeans, just imagining your tongue stopping the stream short of the absorbent denim.

Stop dreaming. Go for it. You probably don't even have to do a whole lot of talking about this. Try to get at the body parts you want, and your partner will either let you "in" or not. If he stops you from putting your face in his pit, beg or try for another area. In the case of armpits, he may just want to save you the unpleasant experience of getting a mouthful of deodorant. If that's the case, he'll probably remember not to wear any when he sees you in the future. If he lets you get at it, go for it *his* way. Watch his reactions and try to heighten them. If pressure or teeth or gentle stroking get him high, do a lot of that, keeping your attention on his pleasure. If you're lapping at a guy's pit thinking only of how hot it is for you, you're in trouble. You could come up for air and find that he's doing his income tax calculation, trying to ignore you, or trying to pull away from your rambunctious slurping.

On the other hand, if you do what you can get away with in whatever way keeps your man purring, moaning, ordering you about, or reacting in any way, you win and so does he. And that is what good sex, especially good leathersex, is about: mutual pleasure.

While no one would contend that all men arrive in the playroom equal–age and experience, at least, make a difference–it is clear that most men come pretty much similarly equipped: Two feet, one dick, eyes, balls, armpits in pairs, etc. This all adds up to your basic male creature, often a very desirable thing to have around. Then come the toppings and decorations, things which are largely in the power of the wearer to change. We're not talking about clothing, quite. It's shaving or whiskers, muscles or unpumped musculature, body fat or trimness, tattoos and piercings or unmodified skin.

What happens with a lot of beginners in leathersex is that they create, from the self-expression choices made by their first Top, a menu of fetishes. If the man who brought them out to leather/SM was bearded, gym-built but now sporting a gut, with tattoos and a piercing in his dick, the newcomer becomes obsessed with that exact combination, closing the range of possible play partners to a ridiculously narrow band of options. Warning Number One: Don't do this. Warning Number Two: Don't overlook the possibility that you actually do have an effective erotic fetish for one or more of your first Top's characteristics. After all, you found him attractive enough that he was able to do things with you no one else had ever done.

Confusing? Yes. Chances are that you will have your early leathersex experience with someone not precisely of your choosing. You will approach or be approached by the one or few men you can find who are in the scene in the way you think you want to be. Once you begin to build a network of familiar faces, don't demand that every one of them look like the guy(s) you found easiest to connect with on day one. On the other hand, don't ignore anything that gets you hard, keeps you going, and gets you off.

One important thing to notice is that what a man chooses for himself, whether changeable like shaving or permanent like a tattoo, is necessarily a message about who he is and how he is living his life. Some of these things may change tomorrow or next week, though, and what you see may have a very different meaning to him than it does to you. Don't set yourself up for a fall by becoming overly attached to hair, body jewelry, or other things that may not be there next time you see him (or, for that matter, on another otherwise hot man).

It is worth wondering what the whiskers and piercings, hours in the gym, or pounds around the waist are about, too. Think about what your choices mean to you, to give yourself some idea of what other men's choices might mean to them. The answers can range widely, from making conscious or unconscious efforts to become the man of your own dreams, to doing consistently what gets you the sexual partners you want. Some guys grow whiskers they don't care about one way or the other because they get laid more often with them than without. The same reasoning sometimes attaches to piercings, tattoos, and body hair. Your reasons, or anyone's, for having or not having certain elective details of appearance can include simple facts like, "it's what I have to look like to get by in my career," and "because of what I have to look like all week, I got *this* to show off on the weekend, just for relief."

In the end, without getting personal and specific, nothing is *always* true about the details of anyone's grooming and self-care. And if you want to play with a guy in any way, you need to protect yourself from wanting only his beard, his Prince Albert, or anything else that might change. Wanting to play *mostly* with a man's feet or pits, is a safer obsession. Leathermen may be bearded and unwashed, they may sport beer bellies or spare tires, get tattoos and piercings, grow long hair or shave their heads into mohawks, or go all the way to smooth. If you let any of these things become essential to your idea of what is right for a Top or for any leatherman, you are heading down a dead-end street. Time, your tastes, and even fashion trends change it all, and you can be left with no playmates.

It may seem that too much emphasis is being placed on all of this. You may be asking yourself how any of it could matter so much, but there are plenty of men out there who are still so attached to the details of the clean-cut but rebellious, leather-clad, discreetly tattooed icon of the Brando-esque '50s that they sit alone moaning that there just aren't any "real leathermen" around any more. And, in the 1990s–as in every clump of years–another image of the rebel is emerging. This one has wildly eccentric hair, big tribal tattoos, multiple piercings and loves his "bad-ass attitude," but this young man is no more the "real leatherman" than the Brando-clone was.

The idea is to keep your options open. Enjoy what comes along. *Behave* obsessively about mohawk haircuts or soft bellies or whatever does it for you if you want, but don't let anything visible become your definition of what is real or right for a Top, a man, or a leatherman. The stuff that makes the man comes from inside. It's who and how he is that matters, not the ways he landscapes his appearance–which is no excuse for not enjoying the landscaping.

DRAMATIC FANTASIES

If acting on your fetishes is pleasurable, having your fantasies fulfilled can be an earth-shattering way of playing with pleasure. Some fantasies, of course, involve pain, but many do not. Still, most of the fantasies that are not acted out regularly are kinky enough that they are more likely to be well-received in leathersex circles than anywhere else.

Acting out your fantasies in a leathersex scene can be deeply satisfying. The possibilities are endless, and it seems that there is a partner or group for every possible fantasy. For some people the fantasies to be acted out are sex acts or fetishes they have yet to experience in the reality of their sex play. To act on these things is no more complicated than *doing it*. It can be as simple as offering your dreamed-of sex act or fetish to a partner, joining a group of men who are devoted to the body part or toy that is your fetish, or going to the party established to serve people who share your desire.

If your fantasy is a dramatic scene, something where two or more people take on roles and stay with them through the sex play, it is a little harder to set up, but still no problem. The important thing is to have the courage, even the audacity, to go for it. You're not likely to find a gladiator to play opposite your bath boy or an innocent convict as the counterpart to your hardened criminal if you never put the word out that you're ready to play.

We deny ourselves enough these days, often for good reasons. But there is no excuse for denying ourselves sexual pleasures for no other reason than that we're afraid of being misunderstood, laughed at, or rejected. Expect all of that when you go shopping for players, although serious leathermen are more likely than other gay men to listen and either cooperate or not without putting you down. If and *when* you are turned down, realize that it only means you have approached the wrong person. It is the scene that has been rejected, not you. And, of course, this means that you would not have gotten what you wanted with that person anyway. Be glad that you were turned down from the start rather than disappointed in the scene.

Finding someone to share and act out a fantasy is one of the few situations where networking among your leathersex acquaintances can easily fail. Nonetheless, try this route first. If no one turns up who is into your special scene, don't give up. You still have two obvious and viable choices, three counting the possibility of hiring an "escort" to act the necessary role.

First, you can advertise. Usually, personal ads are not a particularly good way of meeting leathersex partners, but the situation may warrant the extra effort involved in sorting out safe and unsafe respondents. You can get past the problems inherent in connections made through personal ads by just getting to know your respondents in several meetings before you get into a sexual situation that might be dangerous with a stranger. For the sake of a treasured fantasy, the time spent will be well-invested anyway, but you might end up with the bonus of a lot of new friends whose tastes at least border your own.

A few last words about personal ads: Be specific and make your statements in positive terms. Write "Wanted: muscular Latino pirate of any age to abduct trim African tribesman, 34, for weekend." Don't write "Ethnic man wants extended fantasy bondage scene, no fems, no fats, no whites."

Then there is the other option. When networking doesn't net the results you want, and advertising either fails or doesn't appeal, you can negotiate for what you want. The basic idea is that you can almost surely find someone else in your network of acquaintances who has role-playing fantasies he'd like to work through. If so, make a trade. Be the jailer to his inmate in exchange for him playing AWOL Marine to your Military Policeman. If at first you don't succeed, broaden the negotiating circle. Three men, for instance, might be able to barter themselves into couples and/or three-ways that cover everybody's fantasies.

Imagine, for instance, these three men: Bud, a black man, wants to be a slave for a cruel plantation owner. Will, an older white man, wants to capture and interrogate a prisoner escaping from his concentration camp in Nazi Germany. Gary, a young blond, has a fantasy about being the Senior bottom, passing on to a "novice" bottom whatever the Top does to him. (These are real people and real fantasies from among my real friends.) Will can play plantation owner for Bud. Bud can play "novice" bottom with Will and Gary. Gary can escape from Will's concentration camp. (This series of scenic options is pretty much what the guys were doing at the time of this writing.) Everyone gets what he wants.

The one overarching rule of fantasy sex scenes is simple: If you don't ask, it won't happen. That applies for all sorts of nonfantasies, too. If you're eager to get into bootlicking, armpit servicing, body worship, genital torture, or any other special sex act, you have to put your ego on the line a bit. You have to ask for what you want whether you're looking to be the Top or the bottom in the scene . . . and the satisfaction really is worth the "risk."

TICKLING AND SOFT TOUCHES

One possible definition of torture is too much of anything administered to one person by another. A single jolt of electricity hardly qualifies as torture, but after a few more jolts, everyone would agree that the word applies. That way of thinking is easily understood if the stimulation being applied is electricity, but it is no less true when the stimulation is tickling or light rubbing.

Tickling, especially foot tickling with the subject tied down, can carry the bottom from laughing to squealing to screaming and crying in a very short time. Soft, light rubbing of the body can work the same way. Some leathermen who are into tickling and rubbing only use it up to the point that it stops being pleasurable, or perhaps a little beyond that point. Others carry it to the limit whenever they can.

As play with pleasure, tickling and light rubbing can be a tremendous way to heighten all sensitivity, turn on all receptors, and put a person into a nearly ecstatic state before any actual pain-pleasure or torture per se begins.

Light rubbing over a large area can go on for several minutes, sometimes more than half an hour, and remain entirely soothing. Tickling as a pleasant sensation may not last as long. Either can be extended for a longer time by expanding the area being stimulated, by short periods of inactivity, or by switching back and forth between pointed tickling and soothing rubs. If the right pattern of rests and action, tickling and rubbing can be found, this scene can last for a long time and be very satisfying for both partners. (Interestingly, bottoms can frequently get away with tickling or rubbing Tops, right up to the point of torture.)

If the scene is meant to be pleasurable, only a relatively low-level power exchange in required. With the addition of bondage, other painful stimulation, or special activities in the rest moments, a higher level of trust and connectedness is called for.

One Top in Colorado likes to keep rubbing scenes going for hours. To do this, he works in all kinds of other fetish and fantasy material. Among his favorite added trips are switching between studded gloves and bare hands for the rubbing, pissing all over the bottom's body from time to time to "lubricate" the rub, and having the bottom very, very slowly roll across the floor as he works his magic all along the body as it is exposed by the rolling. More bottoms come back for this abuse than he is able to handle.

BENEFICIAL SM

There are bottoms who are less devoted to pain than they are to feeling good. This is not meant to be a mysterious statement. They want to feel good in the way that they do after a completely successful pain scene, a heavy flogging for example, but they want to get to this feel-good state by what Scott Smitherum called "beneficial SM."

What is beneficial SM? It can be rolfing and other forms of deep tissue pressure, applied by a Top who knows how to find the points at which energy buildups have created nodes in need of attention. It can mean having the Top walk on the bottom's back, or roughly massage the soles of his feet. It can be any sort of health-inducing activity delivered by a Top who keeps his Top attitude in place, meaning the power exchange is functioning throughout the scene. Many bottoms who want this kind of health treatment from Tops, in a scene, cannot bear the same treatments if delivered instead by a practitioner of the specific therapy involved. This becomes at least a few stages stranger when you discover that a man who is a leathersex Top *and* a deep tissue massage therapist often has to identify himself as a Top and *not* as a therapist to get one of these beneficial SM scenes going.

The number of possible play styles under this heading is hard to determine. Piss drinking as Urine Therapy might qualify for some guys. Postural demands that others might call torture could fall into this category if the postures involved are from the Alexander Technique's ideology or from hatha yoga. Suspension bondage, inversion bondage, and forced calisthenics are all activities that fans have been known to tolerate as beneficial SM. All kinds of habit control, attitude adjustment, and physical therapy can qualify if, as with the rest of leathersex, the partners agree to the definition.

PLAYING WITH THE PLEASURE OF SEX

Given an overlay of bondage or some other element from the typical leathersex repertoire, any vanilla sex act can be part of a leather or SM scene. Some ways of handling the sex drive itself, however, are pure leathersex in and of themselves.

Milking comes to mind in this connection. To milk a guy means to make him come, then make him come again, then again, until ecstatic sensations and orgasms turn into torture (referring to our "too much of anything" definition of torture). Maybe pushing the scene to the point of actual torture moves it out of the range of playing with pleasure, but it doesn't damage the credentials of milking as a leathersex scene. Besides, you can always stop short of torture, and move on to some other kind of stimulation. For some guys, after they have had one or two orgasms, to do anything erotic *at all* will require the full strength of an irresistible Top demanding it, and a power exchange in effect to encourage the bottom to act against his own superficial instincts.

Another way to play with the pleasure of sex in leather is to introduce fetishes to the sex acts. Since body-part fetishes were discussed earlier in this chapter and since acting on them is sex itself, not just an adjunct to sex, the fetishes we are here concerned with are props and materials. That brings leather to mind, but leather is far from the whole story.

LEATHER AND KINKY SOFTWEAR

The leather men wear can sometimes stack up into so many layers that it becomes a barrier under which the men themselves can barely be discerned. The usual answer to this is to organize the clothing so that only the outer layer is leather, leaving the leather shirt home, for instance, when wearing a leather vest or jacket; leaving the vest behind when wearing the jacket, or putting the vest onto the jacket as an overlay. If the point of wearing leather is to look hot, not to roast yourself in a barroom, this answer works.

Then there are leather fetishists, some of whom will gladly roast in their own juices if the oven they cook in is all leather. They like the smell of the leather, and that's usually what they mention first when speaking of it. They enjoy the feel of the leather–either side, as appropriate–on their skin. They feel good thinking of their leather clothing, leather bindings, layers of burdensome leather jackets, vests, overlays, or whatever. Sometimes they wax philosophic about the impenetrable barrier–"even human auras don't show through leather"–or the man-animal connection the leather represents. But, in the end, fetishists wear leather largely because they think they look great in it and because the men they want to be noticed by will think so too.

For all it's thickness and toughness, leather is a body revealing material when the garments made from it are tailored for that purpose. Except for the heavy jackets, that's exactly what leathermen's leather garments usually are tailored for, showing off what they are and what they've got, even exaggerating it. And this is exactly what connects leather and leathermen–whether fetishists or not–with the wider range of "kinky softwear."

It was Mikal Bales, of Zeus Studios' fame, who coined the phrase "kinky softwear" to refer to all the soft and stretchy things leathermen were beginning to wear in the late 1980s. Very likely these nonleather garments and fabrics would never have gotten enough notice to warrant a categoric name if Spandex had not appeared on the scene. With the advent of Spandex (and other skin-tight, super-stretchy, clinging fabrics), there were suddenly noticeable numbers of fetishists praising tights and other clingy clothing, and they were mostly leathermen. So, without especially expecting to see anything, some leathermen looked around for an explanation, and it was right at hand.

Leathermen—beasts of physical appearances, self-assurance, sexual openness, and fashion trailblazers in their way—have long been on the cutting edge in accepting, adopting, and promoting clothing that puts as much body as possible on display. Tight T-shirts and tank tops, jock straps chosen (even dampened if necessary) to be revealing of what they cover, snug-fitting uniforms from just about any source, the various form-fitting and skin-framing costumes of wrestlers, and to a lesser extent even the sleek, painted-on outfits of comic book super heros joined ass-hugging denim jeans along the way. And every addition to the list of kinky softwear has inspired its share of both imitation and fetishism. Leathermen, always remaking their icons and paragons, find many of their purposes well-served by form-fitting clothing.

Most of this Niagara of soft stuff, so helpful in displaying the sculpture of the body, is easily mixed with leather. It is even better than levis in some ways. You can have tighter chaps if they are going over nothing thicker than spandex, or the waistband of a jockstrap.

Whatever it is, if it helps a man to put his sexuality and his virility *out there,* if it helps him make a clear statement about who and what he is, and about what he wants, there will be leathermen who will want it, lots of it, *now.* And, if it is something that leathermen wear, especially if it is something leathermen wear to bars and parties, it will be something that some leathermen (often guys who don't wear the same thing themselves) will find erotically charged. They'll want it on themselves, on their partners, around them in the play space, or even used in stimulating them during sex.

A Top standing over a bottom in tights, with his chaps on or off, turns every curving muscle of his body—not to mention his cock head and balls–into the grapes of Tantalus, especially if the bottom has already discovered the self-torture he can administer by ogling spandex-clad skate boarders and bicyclists. A bottom thrilled by being denied the right to touch the Top's body, can be pleasurably tortured by being forced to massage that body through the thinnest possible covering of clinging, stretchy cloth.

The inner workings of fetishes are the stuff that arguments are made of, but there is no argument among the leathermen who do it about the experience of being driven by a fetish for a particular material, or of manipulating the cravings of a man who is. This can be a major thermostat adjustment, turning the erotic heat to high without necessarily pushing the scene any closer to its orgasmic finale.

Because "leather" is not just a costume or uniform, but a way of being, and a way of being sexual, it can bear all sorts of variations, even variations that don't involve or include the tanned hides of cattle.

Almost certainly, the material most commonly enjoyed by leathermen, aside from leather itself, is rubber. Black rubber garments take all the erotic elements of leather and give them an almost dimensional shift. If leather is form-fitting, rubber is shape-making; if leather is a barrier representing the strength of the wearer, rubber is a dam against which any number of seductions might melt entirely without getting through; if leather connects the wearer to the supernatural man-animal world by being the skin of a powerful beast, rubber connects the wearer to the nature-be-damned world of man as the superior and dominant beast in the jungle called earth. Is it any wonder that rubber wearers tend to be at least part-time fetishists, dedicated to the remarkable capacity of the material to put the merchandise on display, and protect it from any unwanted touch?

When kinky softwear comes into the leather scene, the nonleather materials often bring with them the strange possibility of being entirely on view–curve by curve and detail by detail–as though you were naked, but legally and touch-preventingly clothed.

Naturally enough, leathermen have pushed these new materials to the limit, pressed them into playroom service, and made them "leather." Bondage devices, hoods, blindfolds, gags, mummy bags, and play table surfaces are made of T-shirt knit, Spandex, and just about every material in the kinky softwear category. If the yardage were available, there is absolutely no doubt that whole play rooms would be upholstered in the knit of jockstrap pouches. And, why not? If it adds a single degree to the erotic heat, if it moves the scene a single step toward success, if it touches the cravings or facilitates the joy of a single SM player, is there any excuse for not having it? No. None. What gets us high enough to go on enjoying and caring about our lives and the world we live in serves a tremendous peace-making purpose even if no world leaders will ever know about it.

Chapter Five

Playing with Life and Death

Achieving the most extreme scenes possible is certainly not the goal of SM. Not every player wants or needs to go so far with SM that he can be said to play with life and death. Not every player can. And no one, least of all a stranger writing a book, can recommend playing on the edge to anyone. It's not exactly even a matter of choice for most SM players who undertake the scenes that are often called "playing on the edge." We go, it seems, if we must; and, if we must play on the edge, we will do it, one way or another.

Seeking erotic satisfaction beyond all reasonable assurances of safety and sanity in a physical and psychological arena where the question of consensuality is undefined at best, is as much about challenging the mind and spirit as it is about using and enjoying the body. It can be an intense way to test and expand limits, a way to confirm trust, and a way to risk everything on the hope of transformative ecstacy. For the unprepared adventurer, perhaps striking out in this direction for the wrong reasons, it can be a very dangerous way of playing without limits, regardless of trust, and–because of the psychological attitude implied in a bad approach–almost without the hope of any valuable inner experience.

WHERE THE EDGE IS

Every SM player has his limits. They change over time. They're different under different circumstances and with different partners. Beyond the broad grey area of "most people's" limits, there is a further area where fewer players go, an extent or extreme of pain, submission, surrender, or psychological intensity that is unapproachable for most people. The boundaries of play territory are different for each person, but general definitions are possible. We usually play in the area where the acts and levels of intensity are within the realm of what we consider desirable and likely to be satisfying. This is the realm in which SM is obviously erotic, where we act out our fantasies or discover them. Beyond this is the realm of the fantasies we don't really expect to have fulfilled. One man's "beyond," though, is another's real playing field.

No matter what we say to each other, communication in words is imprecise, barely approximating to the reader or listener what the writer or speaker intends. If the subject is highly personal–say sex or death, danger or fear, transcendence or fulfillment–the communication gets murkier still. There is no way to say what it means to play on the edge. One man's edge is another man's daily life; one couple's far-flung fantasy is another's foreplay. When a man gets his kicks by pushing another man to the brink of coma by depriving him of breath or lacerating his skin in rapid-fire lashes of a whip or strokes of a knife, that is at the very edge for most people, but maybe not so far-out for the players involved.

Still, playing on the edge is something. The phrase means something. And no matter how little we understand each other, we can agree that, for some of us, there is an allure to the edge, the place where pleasure and danger mingle, where ecstasy toys with extinction, where fear and sex and the dreams of the human spirit collide or converge, where sparks of self burn brightly, perhaps winking out in the blinding presence of unknowable otherness.

Playing on the edge is playing with self-extinguishing and self-realization. It is playing with the realization of dreams and the destruction of fantasy. Playing on the edge is going one step further than you are sure you can come back from–one step or ten. And, while an ordinary flogging or electrotorture scene is within the province of most SM players, *the edge*–SM in which the danger of losing life, limb, or sanity is real–is a different kind of psychic space, approached by people in different ways.

EXTRAORDINARY EXAMPLES FROM ORDINARY LIFE

"It makes me feel good," Jose said, "and if I die, I die." He might have been talking about SM, but he wasn't. He was being interviewed about his sport of choice, "surfing" on the tops of Rio de Janeiro's intracity trains. Dodging razor-thin guy lines and bare high-voltage wires, dodging train company security and local police, knowing that about 100 of his fellow "surfistas" die in Rio each month, Jose still climbs atop the trains every day and risks everything because it makes him feel good.

A young ski champion spends more time convalescing and nursing injuries than practicing or competing. Television sports reporter Gary Radnich asks her, "Don't you ever think of quitting and living till you're thirty?" She answers that, despite the major injuries and the "nickel and dime stuff" like broken ankles, she wouldn't consider not skiing because "it's a quality of life question."

Meantime, bungee jumpers say they never feel more alive than in the possibly fatal seconds of free fall as they plunge from a bridge. Sky divers and demolition derby drivers, rock climbers and other athletes in the "thrill maniac" category all echo the sentiment. Life is more life-like, more real, more worthwhile when they present themselves with genuine risks. Not surprisingly, many of the same thrill seekers (and their milder kin who are attached to roller coasters and such) connect the high they get with sexual fulfillment.

Orgasm is the usual metaphor. "It's like an orgasm that goes on forever . . ." "Like the greatest orgasm you ever had . . ." and similar phrases pepper the thrill seekers' descriptions (even if the evening news is a bit shy about running such sound bites).

Orgasm. At "just sixteen," Jose may not recognize what is rumbling under his feet and up through his body as he bobs and weaves to keep alive on top of a speeding train. It's what the bungee cord connects the jumper to, what the methods and instruments of the thrill provide. It's another way of being conscious, one as intense as orgasm, one describable in almost no other than sexual terms. Even joggers, long-distance runners, weight lifters and people who do aerobics know something of this, but they are less likely to speak of it in sexual terms.

The differences between Jose and SM players who go to the risky edge of the scene are simple: understanding and honesty. The leatherman *knows* he is playing with his very existence, challenging and changing its meaning. He admits this, even to himself. To Jose the great challenges are avoiding the cops and staying alive to "surf" again.

GETTING PERSONAL

When my boy–already breathing the thin, used air inside a hood or past the obstruction of my mouth against his–feels my hands constricting his throat, we sail together past the mileposts of trust and consent. We are at least touching the brink of that grey area between ordinary life and actual death. Each of us takes from our play on the edge what he can, and it's usually too much connected to our separate individualities to be easily or comfortably discussed. Nonetheless, we know we have been at the edge, relying on each other and whatever resources we have. We know we have bared our souls completely to ourselves, somewhat to each other, and at least slightly to the Powers That Be in the universe. For a moment or an eternity, Being has become more important than anything we could call knowing or doing or living. At the edge, Being is all. Life blurs and intensifies. Thought dissolves into experienced truth. Wanting and desiring wink out. Liking and disliking are irrelevant. Being is just being, and to *be* is enough. Soul and mind are replenished and refreshed, and–however tired–body is usually left tingling and pleased as well.

We may not see God when we play to the very edge, but *that* is nothing more than a semantic distinction unworthy of discussion. It feels more as though, by pressing ourselves against the flexible edge of existence, we might make ourselves visible to God. (More semantics of dubious value.) The thing that matters is that we see ourselves in a light we could never have known without adventuring to the very heart of danger, and what we see is unforgettable, undeniable, and real.

GETTING SPECIFIC ABOUT EDGE GAMES

The brief paragraphs below–recollections and remarks from a number of serious players–do not add up to a map of the seldom-traveled territories of the leathersex frontier. In fact, they are barely more than snapshots, but they may help you consider where you might like to go, and to know with some certainty where you do not want to go.

Hanging and Strangulation

Breath control can mean breath *limiting*, permitting the bottom fewer regenerative and essential oxygen molecules, less access to the mechanism of internal temperature regulating, but in extreme scenes it becomes something entirely different. Breath control is purely a game of trust, kept entirely between the Top and the bottom. One trusts. The other plays with the limits of that trust to invoke fear, or to draw back from fear, to demand greater trust or to demonstrate his trustworthiness, and to take control of his partner's sense of time in an effort to inch him forward toward the dividing line between time and eternity.

Then, beyond breath control are the fantasies of strangulation and hanging. He touches your throat, maybe even applies a bit of pressure, and you rage. You thrash and get high on the threat as much as on the reduced breathing, but mostly you fly on the fantasy of great danger. Beyond such fantasies is the playing field of the few who really want to be hanged or strangled, a scene that only the most carefully prepared Top can provide, and only the most fully receptive bottom can enter into safely.

"Hanging," says one edge-player in an astonished, but very pleased tone of voice. "It's scary. Scares me too, at times. You are really giving up all control. It's a tremendous rush, just thinking of stepping off the stool. As soon as you start to float, you're there. Afterwards, you *know* you've really had an out-of-body experience, especially if you've passed out for any time. After . . . then my dick is just raging hard!"

This player whose scene is a noose around his neck and nothing under his feet goes on: "You don't want to die at all, you just want the rush." And he explains, "I didn't choose this fetish. I discovered it early, early, early on. In fourth grade, I just wrapped something around my neck, and I came. I don't know why I happened to wrap anything around my neck. Now, if I'm with someone and he wants to punch me in the stomach, that would hurt, but if he wants to put his hand on my neck, that's different . . . Yes! To me, it's a nice form of domination."

For some players, the fantasies surrounding hangings are very important. Their extreme scene is hanging, but not just the hanging. They have to have a U.S. Cavalry Court Martial, a POW punishment, a criminal conviction, or something of the sort played out to set the scene for the hanging. In fact, if the fantasy is played carefully enough, the hanging sometimes loses its importance to the point that they don't want to go through with it, so a rescue is rigged, followed by whatever is in the interest of the rescuer. Probably the most common hanging fantasy, judging by the erotic fictions, is the cowboy outlaw in the wild west, closely seconded by the good cowboy framed by the outlaw sheriff.

Players who do scenes with hanging are well aware how dangerous their game is. Nor is it a lot safer when they turn from hanging to other forms of strangulation, but danger (controlled to a certain extent, of course) is part of the turn-on. It is in the sense of danger and the reminder of their mortality that some guys find the exhilaration that says "life" in the loudest way.

Flogging

Ordinarily, whipping and flogging would not be thought of as playing on the edge. Ordinarily, they are not, but the possibility is always there to have a scene, especially a pain scene, intensified and continued until it carries the bottom (and, at best, also the Top) to the far reaches of the known psychological universe.

The first time I was seriously whipped, almost the first time I even saw floggers and whips, I knew I was not safe. I didn't have any concept of whether what I wanted, and was finally getting, could be called sane or not, but I knew that it was necessary, for me. And there was no discussion that could have been called "getting my consent." I was there, at an SM play party in the 1960s in Los Angeles, and I had been presented to the other players as a bottom. Therefore, I was available for whatever the experienced and mutually accepted Tops wanted to do with me. Consent to their wishes was considered a foregone fact; it was tacitly accepted as universal. I had accepted that I was not allowed to speak unless specifically asked to do so by an authorized Top, so the thought of protesting never occurred to me.

I might now disapprove of those conditions for my own play-room, but they were the rules of the game at these parties for as long as I attended them. What's more, I am glad things were exactly as they were–then and there.

That first real whipping went on and on. I very quickly passed the point at which I could simply resist the pain, and I had no concept of pain processing to work with. Soon I was crying out very loudly, keeping a strand of consciousness always alert against accidentally crying out in words, which would have broken the rule against bottoms speaking. The pain was there at every stroke, taking over everything except my efforts to remain an acceptable guest at the party.

At some point, like a cool rain falling directly from my brain and heart, there began to be spots of painlessness, points of lightness. It was as though the pained, suspended boy of eighteen or so was being left behind, an object barely remembered, not identified with my self at all. Something else, something that I recognized as my-self was being liberated. Like a stamp peeling loose, as the rain-drops of coolness touched me, I floated free.

There was no longer any question of resisting the sensation, that seemed as ridiculous as refusing to feel the warmth of the sun while standing in its light. I worried for a split second that the smile I felt stretching my face might burst out into laughter and stop the scene, but it was a fleeting concern, and I didn't laugh. My body continued to be whipped, intensely but not brutally, as I drifted. It never occurred to me to think of this as an out-of-body experience, but it may be that those words apply. It never seemed quite right to call it a religious experience, although I wouldn't be shy about calling it that today.

Then and there, I discovered that leathersex can lead to trance, to transcendence, and to the deepest and fullest sense of well-being that any physical experience has ever been able to inspire in me. Over the years since, I have discovered that this level of whipping is definitely uncommon. It is playing on the edge and could as easily have led to crisis as catharsis. The Top who presided over this whipping, whose name I didn't even learn until years later, was busy with someone else when the Dungeonmaster's slaves took me down, washed me, and carried me to a bench outside. I have never had the balls to ask him if he knew when he was whipping me that I had never been flogged before. It doesn't really matter. I saw the edge of my life as an inviting abyss, and discovered that–approached this way–it is possible to plunge over the edge and return, changed.

Piercing

Like flogging, piercing is not usually thought of as playing on the edge. When you see the piercings of Fakir Musafar, though, and see how he uses them, you know that there are ways to the frontier with piercing. The inch-plus holes in his nipples and the vertical tunnels large enough to accommodate meat hooks in his pectorals are nothing like ear-piercing, and far beyond what is usually meant by either permanent or temporary body piercings too.

"I've been playing on the edge by piercing my body," Fakir says, "since 1946, when I was 15. The first time I pushed a needle through my skin, I got a rush that was unbelievable. Nobody, but nobody was doing this then." That year Fakir also pierced his nasal septum for the first time. By the following year he was creating his own earliest tattoos, using sewing needles and india ink. More to the point, he also pushed a wooden stake through the side of his chest, attached it to a thong, tied the thong to a tree, and did his first Native American sun dance, a ritual in which the "dancer" pulls at the thong until the skin breaks.

Until he was in his twenties, Fakir's edge play was all done solo, which can turn up the element of danger in many scenes to the point that they become flirtations with death or permanent and unintentional body modifications. By 1955 he was sewing weights to his chest. Starting with 24 small fishing weights, he soon advanced to as many as 60 one-pound weights hanging from fishing lines running through his flesh. In 1959 he gave himself his first permanently installed piercings, in his nipples. These were all major adventures, dangerous games to be undertaken alone and without either support or training, but the play shifted into a higher gear in the early 1960s when Fakir found supportive gay male friends.

With his helpers, Fakir was able to fulfill his dream of experiencing the Kavadi, a frame used in Hindu ceremony with up to 100 sword-like rods held in place around the body, all their tips piercing the Kavadi-bearer's skin at the same time. With the advent of helpful friends, there also came the need to think differently about the dangers he was facing. Suddenly, acting out his dreams required that Fakir sign nonliability waivers covering his helpers in the event of his injury or death.

Friends and waivers in place, Fakir soon also did his first hanging from piercings. The first one used stainless steel wires pushed through his chest muscles, and the hanging lasted for several minutes. By the following year he had a chance to hang "as long as he could stand it," which turned out to be the beginning of his most famous edge game, the O-Kee-Pa. In this Native American ritual, the "dancer" is lifted off the ground by hooks in his chest and ropes that are tied high in a tree. The now-permanently open vertical piercings in Fakir's chest make the insertion of the flesh hooks easy, but there is nothing easy about hanging by the pectorals. (This, by the way, is the ritual that Richard Harris acted out in the movie *A Man Called Horse*.)

"Through all this playing on the edge with piercing, I not only got erotic turn-on, but early on it lapsed over into altered states," Fakir says. He remembers many out-of-body experiences in great detail and understands completely the state of his body left hanging in a tree while he is "out."

"If it is death," he says, "then death be it . . . the benefits are too great to pass it up." He closes the subject very elegantly with, "Dangerous, but significant."

Fire

There is nothing unusual in leathersex circles about guys who like to have burning cigars, cigarettes, or matches held near or pressed into their skin. Heat as stimulation is understandable, a reasonably predictable variant on striking or clamping as stimulation. On the other hand, some people like their fire more raw, more flamboyant than the glowing tip of a cigar.

Fire is powerful both as a physical force and as an image. It's the stuff nightmares are made of, and it touches people in mysterious ways. This is true even if the fire is burning only trees thousands of miles away, and we're seeing only the television report. Even at that distance and at that technological remove, fire can fascinate. Some players, like Raelyn Gallina, close the gap between the fire and the viewer *completely* by putting the flames directly on the body.

It is impossible to describe the effects that are unleashed when flames begin dancing on your skin. There is no substitute for personal experience with this–or any–edge game. The combination of fire as the object of primeval fear and fire as the provider of direct sensation takes the player to the edge fast. "With the element of fire," Raelyn explains, "you always have the elements of chance, chaos, and destruction at a split second's notice. Fire is such a passionate element!"

In SM play, the actual period when the fire is burning on a bottom's skin is usually only seconds at a time, perhaps up to five seconds, perhaps repeated many times and moved around on the body. "But with fire on your skin," Raelyn says, "five seconds is a long time. People reach their limit . . . that wall of fear where they think they're really going to burn. You're dealing with reflexes. You have to be really present there, ready to end it. Fire is playing on the edge for the Top and the bottom, but the edge that the Top rides on, control, is different from the edge that the bottom rides, fear and actually burning."

Psychological Terror

Here's the scene: It's a torture contest at an important SM run where many of the most experienced players gather annually. The bottom has been given a piece of information. The Top's job is to get that piece of information within an alloted time period. The Top sends the bottom off to break a given number of beer bottles–no questions asked–and bring back the jagged bottom halves of the bottles that can still be stood upright. Then the bottom is wrapped in a couple of layers of fish net and suspended from a frame in such a way that his body hangs scant inches above the sharp, upward-pointing broken bottles.

The contest judges come by and announce that the scene cannot be allowed, the Top will have to be disqualified. But the Top persuades them that torture is torture is torture, and is allowed to continue. When the bottom, more than a little shaken that his situation frightened even the very knowledgeable judges, will not give up the essential bit of information, the Top snips through one of the fishing lines. The bottom feels his weight shift. That's real. He feels the sharp edges of glass below, thrusting hungrily up toward his skin. That's the beginning of terror.

The bottom begins to bless his grade school arithmetic teachers as he computes to the nearest imagined ounce that 50-odd strands of 12-pound fishing line can hold X amount of weight. His own body plus the fish nets weigh only Y, so he is safe down to some Z number of fishing line supports–a number that is reached all too quickly, and with the Top always there demanding his attention, demanding the information. Has the Top calculated correctly? What kind of grades did he get in math classes? Is he going to misjudge the bottom's weight or be overconfident about the exact strength of the fishing line, or of his knots for that matter? Finally, there is only one question: Intentionally or not, is the Top going to allow the bottom to drop, with no more protection than a fish net, into a sea of broken glass?

It seems he is. The bottom, being prudent, thrilled, terrorized, past all ordinary states of consciousness, comes to the conclusion that losing the contest is not such a terrible thing. He divulges the secret information. Crash. As soon as the Top hears what he has been trying to get out of the bottom, he slashes the last fishing lines with his knife.

With the force of all his body weight, the bottom falls flat, about eight inches onto the ground. The broken bottles have been removed. The judges' worries were part of the plan. The contest is over, and this psychological terror takes second place to a scene in which breath control and a cattle prod have been used.

"It took me a long time to come down emotionally," the bottom says. "When I was at the breaking point, I was trying to climb out of the net."

Terror scenes are not easily set up in ordinary negotiations between leathersex partners. There have to be cards not shown, points of trust pushed and twisted, surprises and tactics not revealed. No one is going to experience terror–not biochemical-producing, consciousness-changing terror–if he goes into the scene with all the assurances and certainties normally considered basic to safe, sane, and consensual play. It just doesn't work that way. If I ask you to jump out of your chair and shout Boo! at me, I can't really be surprised if you do.

Terror, like fire, is about forces that stretch back into the unrecorded beginnings of human emotions, forces invoked only when we have some concern for our continued wholeness or existence.

OTHER EXTREME SCENES AND CONCLUSIONS

Whenever the subject turns to what is extreme in any sense, it is always possible to imagine what is more extreme. In many cases, when the subject is SM play on the edge, the only possibilities more extreme are death and disfigurement. The important thing to remember in this connection is that a fuller and more fully understood life is the goal. No sane SM player is eagerly seeking death. Nor does anyone want to be disfigured or disabled.

Still, some leathersex scenes are played all the way out to the edge where the danger of never returning or of returning maimed or psychologically damaged is very real. Through power games involving strangulation or hanging, piercing or pain, fire or the relinquishing of all self-determination, some people place themselves at the very fringe of life for reasons only crudely approximated by even the most carefully worded explanations.

No player on the edge wants to unduly encourage you to go beyond your own physical or psychological limits, but some of us cannot resist going. Life itself seems dull when it is unchallenged. To *be* without confirmed Being, to breathe without treasuring breath, to sense without a framework within which to be thrilled by sensation . . . these are all less than we can accept. We want *everything* and we want to know that it is real, so we test all we know, feel, intuit, sense, and *are*. The testing is also growth and awakening. It is, in short, becoming.

Edge players know the dangers of their games. Some of us have even known others who–by going too far, by playing alone when there ought to have been a vigilant Top present, or by some other means–have hurt or killed themselves. We also understand that being too well-known for playing on the edge is a danger. If a man is into hanging, for example, and another man in his city dies by hanging in an SM playroom, who will the authorities call on, and how will an edge player defend himself to a jury? Being known for playing on the edge is an invitation to others, even others in the leathersex communities, to misunderstand and accuse. "It's like being in the closet all over again," one player says, "but you wouldn't believe how many people I correspond with who are into this . . . and they're all closeted about it."

In fact, because of the social dangers overlaid on the physical and psychological ones, many people who take their leathersex play to the edge are known to each other only by pseudonyms. Two men who may know the most absolutely intimate details of each other's sexual and spiritual lives, who go together to the brink of extinction from time to time, often don't have each other's phone numbers. They know where and when they are likely to meet, or they can reach each other through answering services or post office boxes, but they don't know each other in the usual sense at all. This may add a welcome element of uncertainty to some scenes, but it is also a symptom of the crippling of the leathersex community by the attitudes of the larger society in which it is a small and unwelcome minority.

For those who feel they must play on the edge, societal pressures to conform to safer standards have no effect. They do what they must for their own reasons. The scenes provide the rush of terror and the high of biochemical euphoria, but that is not the whole story. The thing that is life-changing about visiting the edge on the broomstick of terror is the strength, self-reliance, and peace that well up as we deal either receptively or triumphantly with the risks of the scene and its aftermath. Very likely, the idea underlying all of this is not unlike what young people experience as they learn to drive. There are dangers, real and imagined; fears, primal and immediate; surprises that inspire new and unexpected dangers; and, eventually, there is the confidence and skill of a safe and capable automobile operator. The difference is that there is no social net under the edge player, no encouraging family or fellow students. There is just his need, his experience, and the effects he accrues.

Almost any leathersex scene can be carried to the point where it places the bottom at the edge in his own perception–some, like "castration," dungeon surgery, scenes involving weapons, and the like, do so more easily than others. The edge, you see, is where you find it. Far from the edge is life the way it is. As we move toward less familiar and less lighted arenas of action and being, something else begins to be possible, something born in danger and uncertainty, something that embraces risk with courage, and turns away from fear for the sake of freedom and clarity. That movement, which must always be *toward* something, and never simply *away from* life, can be made by playing with life and death.

Chapter Six

Leather Relationships

Continuing relationships between leathermen come as quite a surprise to most other gay men, just as gay and lesbian unions surprise heterosexuals. Nonetheless, the wearing of the black is no defense against the nesting urge and the associated emotions. Leather, in fact, only increases the number of ways two men might work out the details of settling down together.

Besides choosing to live together, being roommates who may or may not ever have any sexual contact with one another, leathermen enter into many kinds of formal relationships. Master and slave, Daddy and boy, animal and owner, or full-time Top-bottom situations are relatively obvious possibilities. Leathermen also set up housekeeping as lovers, sometimes even getting "married" as near to legally as any gay couple can. All human relationships vary so much from couple to couple that calling any two unions by the same name strains the words we use to label or define them. Leathermen have their own, sometimes extreme ways of straining the definitions.

LOVERS

A lot of people–straight and gay, leather and vanilla–have trouble with the word lover, but there is no better word in general use for two people who are not legally married but who otherwise have the same relationship expected of married folks. For leathermen, perhaps, the word lover has the added unpleasantness of sounding soft in a world constructed on a kind of hardness, having a slightly feminine sound (for whatever reason) in a subculture that tends to masculinize everything.

Nonetheless, there are lovers in leather. Some couples into leathersex, perhaps even the majority of leather lovers, look and act like other gay men, develop their circles of friends among nonleather guys, and live their lives intentionally disassociated from the leather community, its institutions, venues, and public values. This is a near-equivalent of those gay couples who move to rural areas "to give their relationship a better chance," often meaning that they are choosing to reduce the temptation to be unfaithful to one another by reducing to approximately zero the number of gay-identified men they see regularly.

Lovers who do their leathersex in private and live nonleather lives outside the bedroom are missing out on a lot they might take advantage of in the leather community, but their choices are not completely uninformed. In gay newspapers, if nowhere else, they get reminders of the events, trends, and celebrations of the leather tribe with which they are not associating. And, at least occasionally, they can happen in on a leather contest, beer bust, or dance to feel the otherwise foreign or lost camaraderie.

Some couples end up choosing to lead two lives. They have leather friends and vanilla friends, leather weekends and vanilla weekends, even different ways of dressing and of addressing each other in these separate worlds. These people answer any charge that what they are doing is dishonest, unhealthy, or wrong, with the simple assertion that they are allowing themselves the pleasures of both lifestyles.

LOVERS WITH ADDED DIMENSIONS

Sometimes a man discovers his interest in leather after he has found the lover he hopes to spend his life with. This situation could be played out in any number of ways. The new interest could mean the end of an otherwise successful relationship. It could lead the other party in the relationship to find some corresponding level of interest in leathersex, or a tolerance for some leathersexual expression, keeping the couple together and perhaps improving their sex lives. It could lead to a new arrangement for the couple by which one or both parties are not bound to be sexually faithful to the other, a situation that is especially dangerous if one is exploring new erotic territory. Early leathersex experience can often involve powerful transformational effects.

Another answer to the dilemma of a leatherman in a continuing relationship with a vanilla lover is for the leather partner to make arrangements to have his needs met outside the relationship, without otherwise altering the implied contract with his lover. Suppose, for example, a guy discovers he likes to be spanked. Maybe he even discovered it in play with his lover who doesn't want to do it again. He might find he can meet from time to time with another man–in effect establishing a secondary relationship–for the specific purpose of having a spanking scene. After the scene, he goes home to his lover fulfilled and happy, eager to keep up his end of the relationship at home until it is again time for him to meet with his butt-slapping buddy.

The possible permutations of this arrangement are endless, and the number of couples whose relationships are made possible by them is uncounted. One couple in Denver has had a flogger coming in to whip one of the guys twice a month for over two years. They have leather friends, but don't otherwise have much to do with the leather community. When the flogging Top arrives, he and the vanilla lover usually have a drink, talking about the one thing they have in common, the other lover. Then the Top takes charge of his bottom for the evening, flogs him in the couple's garage, and leaves him there to be brought inside by his lover. They don't expect most people to appreciate how this arrangement supports their relationship, so they don't challenge people by talking about it.

Another couple, in New York, has been together for many years, having started out as vanilla lovers and business partners in the early 1970s. They have gotten into leathersex together to some extent over the years, but their tastes are not an exact match. They are, fortunately, a Top and a bottom, but the Top's interest in pain scenes is much greater than the bottom's. So, they maintain their loving relationship, play together when they are pleased to do so, and sometimes bring home another boy who will take the greater pains the Top is eager to give. The bottom in the couple remains in the playroom and continues to get the kind of SM attention he wants without being expected to do more than he wants. Sometimes he even joins his lover, the Top, taking a junior Top role, helping in the stimulation of the visiting bottom.

Finally, another option for lovers who want to continue their relationship even though it doesn't have all the leathersex options one of them wants is simply to buy the services that are needed. In most states, in fact, prostitution is defined by the use of genitals, so it isn't even illegal to pay someone to beat or be beaten, to humiliate or grovel.

Probably the most common result of one lover discovering an unshared interest in leathersex is that the couple breaks up. Even without a lengthy sociological study, it seems the second most likely result is that the other party also discovers a similar interest. This is not as surprising as it sounds. After all the two were attracted to each other, and their mutual, undiscovered interest in leathersex could even have been part of the original attraction.

Leathermen in relationships that are labeled as something other than "lovers," frequently think of themselves as lovers *and more*. This is even true when, at a glance, the style of the relationship would seem to preclude the very concept of love.

MASTERS AND SLAVES

The sometimes brutal interplay between black slaves and their white masters in the antebellum South is the historical context for Master and slave relationships that comes most easily to American minds. For a night or a weekend, even in interracial pairs with either race as Master or slave, leathermen might play with this kind of history as a fantasy, but it has little or nothing to do with continuing Master-slave relationships. Some tales of Roman slavery, again usually only referred to in short-term fantasies, may be closer to the modern reality, but the truth of contemporary Master-slave power exchanges has no exact historical cognate.

There is no better way to grasp the nature of this relationship than to hear from a couple who are living it. The details vary from couple to couple, but Fred and Michel, cofounders of Masters And Slaves Together (MAST), are not atypical. Fred, the Master, has lived in San Francisco for more than 30 years, and has been involved with the leather scene there since the earliest days of The Toolbox, the city's first leather bar.

The following interview was done in the summer of 1989 for *Drummer* magazine. It has been updated and edited, so that references to time and such are accurate for 1993.

Question: How did the two of you meet?

Michel: I lived in New York City until 11 or 12 years ago, then I moved here because the person I had become involved with lived here. It was my first major SM relationship. We (nodding toward Fred) had met then, when I first started coming to San Francisco regularly to see this other person. I suppose we just acknowledged each other casually. Then I moved out here, and that relationship ended in due course. I think it was doomed from the start. Then *we* ran into each other here about eight years ago, and the thing developed from there. We have now been living together for seven years.

Q: Obviously you are a Master-slave pair. Do you accept words like couple and married? Are these accurate too?

Fred: I think they all are, and that is inconceivable to some people. We have told our friends we are lovers, and they are extremely confused. How can a Master and slave have a loving relationship? This is because, in the strict role-*playing* which some people do, there is not the ongoing, loving, interpersonal relationship. We have friends who are very confused by us because they separate their lives into those categories, and they play Master-slave games. They're not *games* in a bad sense. They're positive, meaningful relationships, but their loving relationship or lover relationship is in a separate category. The vast majority of people, even in leather, have some sort of relationship–whether lovers or what have you–and then they get their leather experiences by coming every now and then down for an episode on Folsom or . . .

Michel: Or with friends . . .

Fred: Or at a 15 party (The 15 Association, a San Francisco-based SM club), or what have you. And this doesn't rock the basic relationship when it's not done in secret. It's just that this is an aspect of their lives that they have to experience. We chose to make it full time, the whole thing.

Q: Full time? Still, there must be some way that you signal each other to turn on the full force of the Master and slave roles so that they don't interfere with the accomplishment of everyday tasks.

Fred: It's the other way around.

Michel: I think that, to a certain extent anyway, we don't do that, the switching roles on and off. The hard thing, actually, is remembering when this sort of thing would be entirely inappropriate.

Fred: Like at a bank or something.

Michel: Because of the fact that we live together, we can live "our roles," if you like, all the time. To some extent, I think this makes it a little easier in that we're not deliberately having to switch *on* and get *into* our parts.

Fred: I think the Master relationship, the M-s relationship, is basic to our relationship. It is the thing into which everything else fits. It's not the other way around. It's not something like, "Oh, now it's time," or "We feel like it." We're not playing a Master-slave relationship. That is the basic premise. Cooking, shopping, sex, all those other things that come into it, play into that relationship, but *it* is the basic thing. This makes it a lot easier, and once that premise is accepted, there's really no serious argument. Well, there have been one or two times, three that I can think of, but we reach a point where we won't challenge that basic premise. If that goes, we lose with it the love, the respect, the future, and what have you. This is constantly reinforced by what he (Michel) wears in the house, how we do things together, what we don't do together.

Q: Can you give a totally mundane example of what you are saying?

Fred: Michel never wears clothes.

Q: A house rule?

Fred: It's not even a rule. It's an agreement. It's a desired state. There are times when I don't care if he wears clothes, but I know he doesn't want to. So, it's an agreement that he will not wear clothes, both as a reminder of who and what he is, and also what *we* are.

Michel: What I'd say is that what, at first sight, would seem a relatively minor thing because it becomes routine and normal, is subtle evidence to both of us. Well, we've been living together for seven years, but I'm still aware that I don't have any clothes on. It's become normal, but it's also somehow, strangely there in mind.

Fred: It's all so simple. We don't think of it as a game. It's a sort of natural thing, he doesn't wear clothes, and he doesn't sit on the furniture.

Q: If Michel is always the slave, doesn't wear clothes, and never sits on the furniture, this must maintain the dynamic of the M-s relationship all the time. This makes it hard to see how an argument could ever get started.

Fred: It's because we are two human beings.

Q: Still, how can it happen? You could always just tell him to shut up.

Fred: I don't think I've ever done that. I've never used the relationship as a power trip. Yes, that may be the basic definition of the M-s relationship, but I've never used it as a put-down, or as final "that's the way it is *because*." Although, we agreed on that before we were together. We knew there were going to be those times in our relationship, and we were very "intelligent" and "sophisticated" about it all, very (laughing) psychological. What happens if we have a strong difference of opinion?, we asked before we got together. Well, we'll hash it out. But what happens if we reach the point where we know there is no way we are going to agree? Then we agreed that if push came to shove in those things, then my word would prevail. Again, by definition, it would, but it has never reached that point. I doubt that it ever would reach a point where I would say "you are wrong because of the very definition of our relationship." But look at him [and we do], look, you can see he's wrong, *by definition*. (Laughing) We use a lot of humor.

Q: Humor could certainly be useful when you need to keep a specific moment from becoming heavier than the relationship could bear, but it is also obvious that humor is a significant factor in your personalities too. It would be there, to some extent, in any relationship either of you had.

Michel: I don't know if this will be any use to you, but I can tell you one moment when it (the M-s power dynamic) just fell apart, and both of us were hysterical. The scene was totally demolished. We have a cat, a very sweet little cat, and we've decided that James is really into SM.

Fred: James is a female cat.

Michel: James is a female cat, so the poor thing is confused already. Apparently this had happened previously, but it so happened that it did not come into my sight, but on this one particular occasion, I was kneeling on the floor and he was whipping me. He had commented before about James peering in and about her wanting to become involved and being fascinated by what was happening. On this particular evening, out of the corner of my eye, I could see James' paw. She was sitting there watching, and she was keeping time with him, swinging her paw in time with his whip. I could see this paw come down, and at the same time I would feel this whack across my ass. I think I stifled it for two strokes, then I absolutely fell apart. He knew what had happened. I think this would be a terrible thing for many people. And it is a terrible thing! Most people in SM have no sense of humor about themselves.

Fred: People might think we don't take *it* seriously, but we do take it very seriously.

Q: In a one-night stand, letting a cat blow a scene would be much more important.

Michel: If this happened when you were with somebody for the first time, you'd just met him, that could blow it forever. When it happens to people who've been around together for a while, it's different.

Q: Yes, when you're together for years, perhaps a lifetime, the memory of a humorously blown scene might be more important than the sexual encounter the moment might otherwise have become. Do you think this relationship is for life?

Fred: Well, it's like any relationship. In a sense, it's no different. We just have a different expression or a different mode than other relationships.

Q: And this is a monogamous relationship?

Michel: Basically, I would say. (Looking to Fred for approval.)

Fred: Basically, but with the exception which we have discussed, obviously. You can't separate the relationship from the roles exactly. And, by the definition of the roles, and of the relationship itself, it's monogamous certainly, on both sides in a certain way, but by definition the Master can do what he damn well wants.

Michel: Yes, yes, he can.

Fred: Whereas the bottom cannot. And I think that is understood. (Michel is eagerly nodding and mouthing agreement.) It is agreed upon. And it was understood and agreed upon from the beginning. But, basically, we're both monogamous. Creating and maintaining the relationship has always been primary.

Q: Sounds like you're describing a relationship that could survive all kinds of things that other people would consider breaches of strict monogamy.

Fred: At one point we considered expanding the primary relationship to include possibly even another live-in, and that never happened. I'm not sure it could, but that's not an impossibility.

Q: That is an option which might, under certain conditions, save the relationship one day. Many leathermen might think that if someone else is *that* interesting, or if things get really tough, they can just let the relationship end and move on to the next.

Michel: But I do think that is a factor of age. I felt like that when I was younger. When you're older you know that something worthwhile is worthwhile, and you don't just throw it overboard for peanuts.

Fred: There is also the factor of being in a gay relationship. We don't have the things that are in other people's relationships, and we don't put that kind of value on it, not the same kind of right/wrong value. We don't have the support of family connections, children, financial involvements, legal structures, religious sanction....

Q: These are stresses all gay relationships must bear. Do you think your Master-slave relationship is better able than other gay relationships to deal with these things, or is it all the more difficult?

Michel: I personally think it is more difficult to establish a relationship when there is an SM involvement. For most people who are involved in SM, it is easy to get their rocks off, so to say. They can go out and party like mad all Saturday night, sleep it off on Sunday, and return to their "normal" way of life, another way of life, on Monday. So, to establish a relationship where this is not something that you are going to do for an evening or a weekend, but as a permanent, ongoing thing is more difficult.

Fred: I think it is more difficult to establish a relationship, but it's easier to maintain a relationship when you have, as we do, some parameters, some framework.

Michel: I think, to some extent, the sensuality of the roles of people like us is stimulated in a way that certainly wouldn't be true for the regular couple, straight or gay. There are situations where, in everyday, normal life, you have one person fully dressed, sitting on a chair, and reading the newspaper or listening to the radio or something. The other person doesn't have any clothes on, and is sitting on the floor. Though you're not super-conscious of it all the time, it is a factor, and every once in a while you do become aware of it. So it's a constant reminder.

Q: If Michel doesn't sit on furniture, and you do, doesn't that get a little strange at dinner time? (Fred didn't answer. Instead, he just looked at Michel, tacitly giving him permission to answer the question.)

Michel: I'd say that's an exception. To me, anyway, eating is an important part of life, and I enjoy it. I enjoy entertaining, and I enjoy it when we eat alone. But I think that we don't make a pretense about our lifestyle and what we're doing. And I think, in our case, that would be a pretension and something that couldn't possibly be maintained. Apart from everything else, it would be very difficult to carry on a conversation if one of you were at one altitude and the other at another.

Q: Even the exception is noticed then, giving still further reconfirmation to the roles you have in the relationship. Fred, did you come up through the ranks, as they say? Were you a bottom, then a slave, working up to Top and Master?

Fred: That's the accepted way up, and I think the majority do it, the vast majority do it. In my case, it didn't happen. Early beginnings in leather: That's one of those things you can always look back and identify. I can look back to grade school when both the little boys and the little girls would walk me home from school and carry the books. Then I'd take the little boys, and go out and tie them up. And then, when I first sort of became involved in the leather community–about the time when the Toolbox opened–I was judged by my peers to be a Top at that time. Good or bad, I won't respond to that.

Q: Masters don't have to have been slaves, of course, nor Tops, bottoms.

Fred: I've never known a Top that, under the right circum-stances, could not have been a bottom. I have known many bottoms who could never be Tops.

Q: Some bottoms would rather die than be Tops. Is the relation-ship you have now a finished thing, the way you want it to be, or do you expect it to go through major revisions to survive the years?

Michel: I don't know.

Q: If that is a comfortable answer, then change probably isn't important. It could happen; it wouldn't be threatening.

Fred: I'm not afraid of that. If it changes, it changes.

Michel: I think that inevitably the relationship has changed al-ready over the past years, but it's happened so gradually that we aren't particularly aware of it. And I imagine it will go on changing.

Fred: I expected him to come up with an example, and I was really trying to think of something. Yeah. For the first year and a half, you could almost set your watch by us. Along about 9:30 there would be an expectation of some sort of sexual activity.

Michel: 8:30.

Fred: 8:30, was it?

Michel: Is now.

Fred: And you could always tell because all of a sudden a bottle of poppers might appear "hidden" under the edge of the couch or something. I'd say, "He's telling me something." That no longer happens. There are other ways we can work things out, but it's not every night, obviously. At first, it scared me to see that I was getting tired after just a year or so.

Michel: Don't know why you'd be tired.

Q: What about MAST?

Fred: It was an idea that we had because we do think there is a need. The M-s relationship is not universally successful. In fact, when we started thinking about MAST, I knew of only about four couples in the city that were even attempting it. I knew there were others, many others, and we saw there was a need for a support group. M-s relationships have unique problems. We've gotten let-ters from all over the world since we started advertising MAST. Often they say, "We want this, it's natural to us, but we have nothing to support us." And that was the original purpose, to sup-port each other. For questions, technique, contracts, interpersonal relationships, and for inter-gay relations, because the M-s relationship, you know, is about six or seven steps down the ladder of approval even within the gay community.

Michel: And that's okay with us.

Fred: It's fine. We don't want all that, but general disapproval does limit what you will find around you. So we have found a need, and we are filling it. We have a roster of more than 160 members now, most of them not in couples at this time.

Q: But the name of the organization, Masters And Slaves Together, would seem to suggest that your respondents should be people who mean to have M-s relationships, right?

Fred: Individuals who have chosen M-s relationships as the sexual expression of their lifestyle.

Michel: Of the responses we get, a few are from couples. These say, "Oh, this is what we've been looking for–let's get together." Far more of the letters come from people looking for one or the other, Master or slave. Now, how seriously they want this, and how much is fantasy, is a difficult question.

Q: Fantasies of a Master-slave relationship probably interfere a lot for people who know nothing from experience about the reality.

Michel: Well, we hardly go to bars anymore. We're not really bar people. So we tend not to meet people and get into conversations about this. But before we were together, when I was involved in a relationship that was much more public because this other person I was with was a bar person, I would get into conversations with people who would be envious of me, having this relationship, living this way all the time, but when it came down to reality, it was different. You meet a person who really wants to be a slave, and he wants this relationship. Then, the first time he is told, "why don't you get the laundry done today," it's all over. Doing the laundry, dishes, and cleaning house isn't part of their notion of what this is going to be.

Fred: With all due respect, the gay press–whether it's the novel, short stories, magazines, or whatever–doesn't help much. You know that's all fantasy. . . .

Michel: A major factor in the stories is that, invariably, the whole relationship takes place in a land of make-believe. Everybody has lots of money. Nobody has to do anything sordid like go out and work. Usually, the Master is of enormous wealth, inhabits this vast palatial home, with a dungeon bigger than most people's homes are. They never work. It's just non-stop sex.

Fred: The more you talk about it, the more I like it. Where do I sign up? But, getting back to MAST, it's going to be whatever people want it to be. And one of the things people want it to be is a contact service.

Michel: One thing about it is there are very few of us. The number of people actually living in Master-slave relationships on a day-to-day basis is very small.

Fred: We have participated in the two major SM clubs for men here, The 15 and the Knights Templar, so you would assume we would know, at least by sight, almost anybody publicly involved in M-s relationships in the Bay Area.

Q: Not many to know, eh? [Fred and Michel both shake their heads.]

DADDIES AND THEIR BOYS

Generally, to the extent that the popularity of various fantasies and various topics of conversation can be a guide, it seems that leathersex has shifted its focus in recent years away from rigid Top-bottom and Master-slave situations both in overnight play and in long-term relationships. This is not to say that leathermen don't play this way any more. We do, but less exclusively, perhaps less frequently, and investing less of our identity in the play than was the case in the leathersex communities of the 1950s and 1960s.

The Master-slave arrangement was the epitome of leathersex at one time, the thing people spoke of as being "further along," even by people who had no intention of "going so far." Today, the Daddy-boy relationship is probably the quintessential relationship for contemporary leathermen. (Still, though, the perfect relationship for any two men is whatever they want and are satisfied by!) Personal ads are full of Daddies seeking boys, and boys seeking Daddies. T-shirts printed "Daddy" and "Daddy's Boy" are everywhere. And, the leathersex relationships that seem to last are the ones defined by the participants as Daddy-and-boy, or something of a similar tone.

Some of the attractions of the Daddy-boy relationship are pretty obvious. There is the warmly familiar language, in terms of the words used and the psychosocial postures and nonverbal communications. There is the fact that "straighter" friends who are puzzled or worried by Master-slave situations can actually learn to accept, even embrace a Daddy-boy relationship. And, perhaps most importantly, there is the fact that a Daddy-boy relationship can be built to exact, personal specifications that include an almost endless variety of options.

Men who can be successful Daddies tend not to be people who have a deep need to be perceived as extremists or outsiders in the way a Rebel Biker or Slavemaster is. But then, what it takes to be extreme and outside now is much more than it once was. To wear leather at all in 1959 was to be an outsider of a relatively extreme sort. This was less the case in 1969, hardly relevant in 1979, and not true to any stigmatizing extent in 1989. So the shifting of social acceptance in the gay community and the world has contributed to the redefinition of acts, attitudes, and clothing in such a way as to support–but by no means create–the rise in popularity of the Daddy-boy relationship.

A man who is likely to be a successful boy must share his Daddy's willingness to be in a leather relationship that does not seek outwardly to outrage. This is an important consideration, but it may only be understandable for the people it *dis*qualifies. Many of the men who are looking for Daddies today would once have looked for Masters, but they would then have been the ones who looked forward to the day when they would turn the tables on the Master, Top him, and then (very, very likely) leave him. In times past, regardless of the fact that most of these guys never got around to the table-turning stage, those who did usually ended up with another Master before long. They hadn't changed their needs. What they had done was simply wear down their Masters.

If you want a relationship where the Top is dominant not only "by definition," but also because of his strengths and the admiration the bottom has for him; where there is respect flowing both ways within the relationship; where one party admits to learning and both parties are accepting of growth and change; where the bottom is expected to have a will and to know when to express it as well as when to relinquish it, a Daddy-and-boy relationship is probably just what you want. And there is one more thing that is very usual in Daddy-boy relationships and fairly uncommon in all other leathersex situations: Daddies and their boys are almost always allowed by the parameters of their partnership to affectionately *express* genuine love for one another.

Love may not be uncommon in any human relationships, Master-slave and other rigid Top-bottom affairs included, but what other set of labels can two men apply to themselves which will give them a more perfect framework for expressing masculine love than Daddy and his boy?

As for the power exchange and sexual interaction between Daddies and boys, it can be quite surprisingly flexible. Age is not a determining factor: Daddy may be younger or older than his boy. The words Daddy and boy are nonlimiting labels: Daddy may be the active or passive, dominant or submissive, Top or bottom partner. All of that is open to negotiation and discovery.

Daddies and boys are the only leathermen whose relationship roles are labelled on the basis of emotional rather than physical activity. The word Daddy has a long history, especially among heterosexuals, in the arena of romance and relationships. It implies a sense of security and emotional support coming from the man called Daddy and, not infrequently, financial support as well.

Boy, on the other hand, is a word with a very different history. Everything we can say about the word boy is debatable, uncertain. Its origin is lost in the earliest mists of the European languages; the twists and turns of its etymology are explained in half a dozen or more mutually exclusive ways. In this century, white people have spat the word boy at blacks in hate, then gone home, smiling and glad, greeting a son with, "Have a good day today, boy?"

The following brief interview may shed some light on the question of what contemporary leathermen mean when they call themselves or their partners boys. Scott Smitherum (my boy until his death in June, 1992), in a rather frivolous mood, took a purely boyish approach to answering the questions.

Question: What do you mean when you say you are a boy?
Scott: Being a boy means I have the freedom to play, a safe place

to do it, and a Daddy, which means lots of love and a nurturing relationship with a lot of growth. It means getting to wear silly clothes, and someone else takes the blame for them. It's permission to be silly sometimes.

Q: Does a boy have to be young?

Scott: No. A boy can be any age, which is good for older boys who like young men.

Q: Does a boy have to be childlike?

Scott: No. A boy should have the ability to be childlike when appropriate, but he also has to be able to function as a normal, human, male adult.

Q: Is a boy still a boy when he is not in a relationship with a Daddy?

Scott: Part of being a boy is giving up decisions and, when you're not in a relationship, you can't do that. But, if I wasn't already a boy, how would a Daddy know who I am?

Q: Can a guy become a boy because it's what the fellow he loves wants from him?

Scott: Yes, if he really wants to. Some guys who are called boys in relationship to men who are called Dads will never be boys. You have to truly want to do it. If you want to do it, it adds to your life. If you're *just* doing it to please someone else, it may just cover up something else in yourself, maybe something you really need.

Q: Does a Daddy-boy relationship have to be an SM relationship?

Scott: No, Dads and boys don't have to be into SM at all. What is needed is a strong figure, and someone who wants to be a stronger figure–a Dad and someone who wants to be more like Dad.

Q: Of course there are a lot of couples these days who are in the leather community even though their only leathersex experience, and the only one they want, is the power dynamic of their Daddy-boy relationship. But, if the couple is doing SM, do you think the boy should always be the bottom?

Scott: No, it's all in how the couple defines it. They are the ones living with the contract or agreement.

Q: How is Daddy-boy different from Master-slave as a basis for a relationship?

Scott: Master-slave relationships can exist without love or romanticism, Dad-boy relationships can't. Other than that, a Dad-boy relationship can take you right up to the edge of the Master-slave relationship. But it doesn't have to go that way.

Q: What does a man need in order to be a boy?

Scott: Honesty. A sense of fun. A need for a strong "father figure" in his life even if he has a good relationship with his father, and a desire to learn from and be like "said strong person." Oh, and a good hot butt.

Q: What kind of satisfaction can you get from being a boy, since a boy seems to always be serving someone else's needs?

Scott: You can get the joy of a job well done and the love of a good Daddy. And, really, it works out pretty well if you have the right Daddy. Like, if you don't want to do the fucking, don't want to stick your dick in someone else, you can have a Daddy, and he'll do that for you.

Q: Slaves often have to wear collars. Should boys also wear collars, locks, and things like that?

Scott: Boys should wear whatever their Daddies tell them to, though they are not precluded from trying their own ideas to seduce Daddy. But they should never wear anyone else's collars or locks without Daddy's permission.

Q: What encouragement can you give to a boy who is worried that by being a boy he may be damaging his manhood?

Scott: If you're happy being a boy, and you're a man, your manhood is assured. If you're covering up some part of yourself to be a boy, you may be in trouble. Manhood means you're a functioning human male, and you need that to be a boy.

Q: How did you come out as a boy?

Scott: My search was always for a mentor relationship. My tendency was always to be sort of passive. So, it just developed naturally. It was something to fall into more than it was a coming out.

Q: Is a boy always in "boy mode"?

Scott: No. There are times when Daddy doesn't need me in boy mode, but it's dependent on Daddy's needs, not mine.

Q: What can a man expect from a relationship with a boy?

Scott: Undying loyalty. Woof, woof!

ANIMALS AND KEEPERS

If Daddy-boy relationships are on the gentler and less rigid side of most Master-slave relationships, the harder and more rigid side is the animal and keeper. And, if true Master-slave relationships are rare, animal-keeper situations are far, far more rare. It may not be that unusual for two men to get together for an evening or a few days, and have one of them take the role of dog or horse for that time. When it comes to a continuing relationship, however, animal-keeping is usually a game played for short periods within the relationship, not the nature of the continuum.

Still, there have been such relationships, and there may be a lot more of them than we know since they are hardly easy to pursue in anything like a public way. The intensity of the power exchange between animal-man and his owner/keeper/trainer would burn out any ordinary human personality in short order, but there are men who will settle for nothing less than that fire.

In this relationship, the bottom is a beast, usually denied the use of his hands, denied the right to stand erect, denied the right to speak in words or even show any more than a dog-like comprehension of human language. Long periods leashed, chained up, or caged are usual, and cannot, in any case, be complained about by any nonanimal means. Punishments are frequently very severe when an animal behaves badly, and even when he doesn't recall doing anything worthy of punishment.

Since people keep animals—the born four-legged kind—supplies and equipment for animal-owning relationships are readily available. Human-tailored equivalents are relatively easy to come by as well because of the number of short-term leathersex encounters based on the animal-owner model.

An animal and owner relationship carries immense psychological risks, like those attached to the worst kinds of humiliation and verbal abuse. It sets up parameters of physical interaction that can be very accommodating of injury and uncontrolled brutality. And it basically means the bottom has no human life of his own. None of which disturbs the few hearty souls who cannot be satisfied with anything less than complete abasement, total destruction of their dignity, and the eradication of their wills. What's more, of the three postrelationship animals I have met, all were sound, sane, reasonable men after from one to four years as beasts. One had prepared completely, putting his assets into an interest-bearing account that was waiting for him when his animal years came to an end. The others were left scrambling and needed help to get back on their feet. (Pardon *that* pun.) And all were still in awe of the powers of their beastmasters, nostalgic for the special sort of dignity they discovered in becoming perfect animals, and ready to go for it again.

Becoming a boy seems safe enough, barely different in degree from being the more passive lover in any gay relationship. Slavery is a bit more dangerous for weak men, but it attracts those who need it, and usually repels those who enter it by mistake. The animal condition, though, is probably most attractive to the people least able to bear the intense shift of psychological and spiritual reality it entails. Fortunately, it is so hard to maintain in the beginning that it is simply unattainable for most of those who approach it, which provides a sort of automatic safety valve.

FAMILIES AND STABLES

After the group marriage experiments of the 1960s, a few of which have survived into the 1990s, most people, gay and straight, returned to the idea that relationships worked only in groups of two. Leathermen were experimenting with relationships for parties of three or more long before the 1960s, and many of those experiments have proven successful.

Just about any leathersex relationship can be extended to include one or more additional people. A Master can certainly be served by more than one slave, and–despite Biblical injunctions to the contrary–a good leather slave can also serve two Masters. A Master with a stable of slaves is more common in fiction than reality, but it happens, and it works. A family made up of a Daddy and several boys is relatively common these days, and there are a few lucky boys with two Dads.

Still more complex group arrangements also exist, some of them lasting for many years, despite the remarkable stresses on all relationships in the age of AIDS, personal ads, computer bulletin boards, and publicly advertised leather bars.

Many group relationships start out as more typical Master-slave, lover, or Daddy-boy households. With the addition of another bottom, the relationship opens up. After that, if one or another of the members of the household becomes interested in someone outside the family, the easiest way to deal with the new affair is to accept the new man into the household.

Almost predictably, one result of letting the family grow in numbers is that the family's sexual repertoire changes too. Some originally leathersex families end up with nonleather members. Lovers who never worked out anything like an agreeable leathersex relationship—two bottoms, for instance—sometimes solve their problems and stay together by adding a leatherman to their family.

Whatever combinations of bottoms, Tops, and their lovers you can imagine has probably happened by now somewhere. And the good news is that experienced leathermen, their honesty and trust trained by the pressures and necessities of safe, sane leathersex interplay can often make these arrangements work.

One family history will suffice to suggest how malleable the leathersex family can be. In this case, the beginning was a couple of vanilla lovers who slowly discovered mutually satisfying leathersex interests. Then, after a number of years together, the Top began to go out, and found another bottom he wanted to add to the household. Never imagining that he'd cash in the voucher, the bottom accepted the new boy into the household on the condition that, if he ever happened to fall for another Top, that man could also join the family. A year later, the family was two Tops, in separate houses a few miles apart, with the two bottoms, now serving as slaves, shifting back and forth between the houses on orders. Within the next year, one of the Tops found himself a vanilla lover, and moved him into the house. Special arrangements were made about his very strictly limited dependence on the slaves, but all remained stable.

Now, three years later, both Tops and one of the slaves have vanilla lovers. The other slave also serves a few days a month in the house of a third Top who uses him extensively as a party decoration and "public toilet." Everyone is very happy (most of the time) and the whole family meets together only once each three months for a meeting at which all roles and ranks are dispensed with during the opening "bitch session."

MAKING A SUITABLE CONNECTION

What kind of man are you looking for? What kind of relationship do you want? What kind of leathersex do you feel is right for you? These questions are very closely related, more intimately interdependent than they are for your vanilla brothers. If you are hoping for a relationship that lasts more than a few hours, you need to know and be able to talk about your sexual interests and your intentions for the relationship with the same confidence you bring to ordering breakfast in a familiar restaurant. (Of course, people survive mistakes all the time. You will, too, many times probably.)

Relationships can be as different as the people who enter into them, and–Top or bottom–you have to be willing to face the ground rules of whatever relationship you get into gladly, or you're "doomed." So, go easy, go slow. Get the experience you want, taste whatever supposedly forbidden fruit you're thinking you might just like. And, eventually, if Mr. Perfect shows up, get into the relationship you want, but make it a realistically defined one, for yourself and Mr. P. Getting into a leathersex relationship, then trying to change the partner or the partnership to suit yourself might work sometimes in vanilla romances, but it can be much more difficult, even dangerous in leathersex relationships.

Chapter Seven

Anatomy, Physiology, and First Aid

The more you know about the human body, the more effectively you can torture and stimulate it. Similarly important, the more you know about it, the more *safely* you can work it over. Tops need to know something of the geography of nerves and muscles, tendons and ligaments, bones and organs in order to stimulate without injuring bottoms. Bottoms need to know, too, so they can be comforted by their understanding or appropriately alarmed, and so they will feel sure of themselves when they permit a specific act or avoid one.

ANATOMY

The rules of nature, including "the survival of the fittest," have produced modern humans who are able to bear a great deal of being knocked around. The vital organs are mostly housed safely within the skeleton. Important nerves and blood vessels are mostly either embedded in or behind muscles, or placed in deep channels, such as the armpit. The skeleton itself is reinforced at its otherwise most vulnerable points with shields of muscle. And the muscles are largely protected by virtue of their capacity for relatively speedy recovery from trauma.

Relatively light SM with healthy men, then, is generally safe with ordinary levels of mutual responsiveness and reasonable caution. No special knowledge, beyond common sense, is required for the lightest and briefest scenes, but very few people are willing to remain within such restrictive limits.

The body can be described as a complex system of facilitating tools and protective mechanisms dedicated exclusively to the use of

167

the person it houses. Of course, a complete study of all those tools
and mechanisms would easily be the work of a lifetime, and even
though perceptive leathersex players are constantly learning, a lifetime would be too great an investment to undertake before playing
at all. What follows here is not meant to be anything more than the
most rudimentary primer. It is a starting point from which you will
be able to combine your play with further learning, on the basis of
which you will be able to determine what additional information
you need for the kind of SM you are going to pursue.

The Head and Neck

The skull protects the brain, but even with a thick mane, it is slight
protection for such a preeminently vital organ. Generally speaking,
except for the sexual use of the mouth, some face-slapping, and
carefully fitted hoods, gags, blindfolds, and head harnesses, the head
should simply be considered off-limits for leathersex. (If you want to
play with someone's head, use words and visual imagery to play with
what's inside rather than risking damage to the skull.)

The mouth and jaw can be injured by rough play, but the likely
problems–abrasion, overstretching, and bruising–will be obvious.
So, to the extent that it is desirable, these things can be avoided.
Less obvious and more complicated is disalignment of the tempo-
ral-mandibular joint (TMJ). A lot of people suffer tremendously
from TMJ problems, but it's almost never initiated in the leathersex
play space. Those people who know they have the problem should
not allow anyone to slap them, fuck their faces roughly, or stretch
their mouths open.

The neck is a vulnerable point. Vital blood vessels between the
heart and the brain pass along the length of the neck. Breathing
passages are located in the neck. The least supported segment of the
spine is found in the neck. While a well-trained and experienced
Top can manually close down the air passages for a certain amount
of time, and the flicking of a few not-too-heavy whip tails on the
back of the neck will not cause any actual injury, this is not generally a safe area of play. In fact, Tops who doubt their ability to land
every whip stroke where they intend, or who are playing with a
bottom who might move between strokes, should seriously consider

putting a heavy posture collar on the bottom to protect the neck during a flogging.

For many bottoms, the mobility-impairing effects of a posture collar heighten the sensual enjoyment of the scene. Others will be frightened by the sensation. If the bottom cannot easily bear the feeling of a posture collar, similar safety can be provided (although with a less desirable visual effect) by draping a large towel or a pair of jeans around the bottom's neck, leaving the ends hanging free down the chest. A leather vest can be used as well, but it will be harder to keep in place.

The Torso

For the most part, the torso is the playing field. From the shoulders to the crotch, there are large areas that are safe for most kinds of SM. Arms, legs, and their joints; genitals, anus, and the joints of the crotch are not included here as parts of the torso.

From the back, the torso is basically a safe zone for play, with the single exception, anatomically, of the waist area, and the possible exception, technically, of electrical toys. At the waist, the spine is not in a muscle channel as it is higher on the back, nor is it as completely locked in position by either muscles or other bones. This presents the likelihood that strong blows could result in disalignment or other injuries. Fortunately, the mechanics of the Top's shoulder joints and the protruding bulge of most upper backs make it very unusual for a Top to whip or strike the weaker low-back area when the bottom is standing. Besides, blows to the lower back are almost never experienced as pleasure or anything that can be processed into pleasure.

The other danger in the same area comes from the fact that the kidneys extend below the protection of the rib cage. They can be seriously damaged by heavy blows, and may even be hurt by relatively light blows that are repeated long enough. Again, if the Top is unsure that he can control the location of every blow, he should provide protection for the bottom's kidneys. A heavy leather kidney belt, or a standard weight-lifting belt serves this purpose very nicely. Also, a good belt can be fitted with D-rings in such a way that, while protecting the kidneys, it also provides a means for the Top to secure the bottom safely in place, reducing the likelihood that the bottom will jerk or shift suddenly, destroying the Top's careful aim.

On the front of the torso, the collarbones are fairly exposed, just under the skin, flanking both sides of the throat. Any bone near the surface like this presents two kinds of dangers. First, it could be fractured or broken by a heavy blow, although the collarbone is not a very likely (nor a very erotic) place for a heavy blow. Second, the light covering of tissue over the bone could be damaged by a blow that would be safe to the bone.

Just south of the collarbones is the chest, including the nipples. This is prime territory for just about any kind of play, again possibly excepting electrical torture. Judge realistically the amount of muscle here, and go for it. Extremely heavy blows, of course, can still fracture ribs, jar and disturb the heart, interfere with breathing rhythm, cause trauma to the liver, or go astray—the collarbones and face are nearby, as are the less-muscled ribs and the soft belly area. But the chest itself is tough, relatively well muscled, and strongly reinforced by the ribs and sternum.

The ribs below the chest are superficial bones and should only be tortured with restraint. Even light tapping that goes on for a long period can eventually fracture a rib. Consider this area, and all lightly covered bony areas to be better for abrasive torture than striking play.

Sometimes a swollen spleen or liver can be especially susceptible to injury when the chest area is played with roughly. With extreme swelling, they can even press into the space between the lower ribs or extend into the area below the ribs. If the bottom is having any organic pain before the scene begins, play carefully (if at all), and avoid jarring or striking the chest or upper back.

Below the chest is the unprotected belly, the gut, the abdominal cavity. Even though some guys like gut punches, and some are muscular enough to take heavy punching if they are tensed in preparation, this is not a reasonable area for novices to play in. Abrasion may be safe, but generally, it is more reasonable to play with the gut from the inside out (fucking and fisting) than to involve the gut much in externally applied SM play.

The Arms and Legs

The limbs and their joints are easily injured, but not necessarily off-limits for careful players. Nonetheless, except with training, it is best to avoid the shoulder joints and armpits, the knees and ankles, and the creases of the crotch with any play except surface stimulation. Tendons and ligaments are bundled in these areas, major blood vessels come to the surface, and some nerves are near the surface and even wrapped around bones at and near the joints.

The major muscles of the arms and legs are relatively safe for most kinds of play, so long so the play does not run the risk of bone fractures. So, for instance, if you have your boy's arms tied straight down at his sides, you would have little concern about a flogger wrapping around his arms a bit, but a baton or single-tailed whip thrown with much force could be a problem. In any case, if you were going to beat or flog a guy with his arms tied down his sides, you'd be wise to put elbow pads on him before tying him up. This way you don't have to be as concerned about hitting his "funny bone," which is actually a nerve bundle wrapped against the bones of the elbow.

There is another danger that is often spoken of in SM circles, even if no one seems to know anyone who has actually encountered the problem. That is, it may be possible to stimulate biceps, calf muscles, or even larger thigh muscles so intensely that they will react with strength enough to wrench a joint or break a bone. This seems highly unlikely, but one wonders how it could be so much mentioned by experienced players if it is completely impossible.

The Hands and Wrists

Hands are, in effect, glove-shaped bags of bones, nerves, and tiny muscles. Except for the simplest and most superficial treatment, it is wise to leave them out of the scene. They may be put into mitts of various kinds to turn them into fingerless paws, and leather shops often have toys specifically designed for this purpose. They may be used as signaling devices, or placed under orders not to move, but it is seldom appropriate to hit, squeeze, pinch, or otherwise torture hands. The opportunities for lasting damage are just too many. On the other hand (oops, pardon that pun!), many Tops find and give a certain sort of leathersex pleasure by placing temporary piercings in the webs between the fingers or by warming the hands with blow dryers or heating pads until the discomfort moves into the range of torture. The safety of scenes including these activities is entirely a matter of the knowledge the Top has about the anatomy of the hand.

The wrists are often tied with ropes or otherwise bound to restrain a bottom in leathersex scenes. There are two categories of danger to this area, both very easily avoided. First, there is the danger of putting too much pressure on the nerves serving the thumb (or, in extreme cases, the whole hand) with overly tight bindings or with bindings that have knots or thicknesses in the wrong place. To avoid this danger, use restraints that hold without squeezing (especially on the area from the side of the arm to the center of the palm, just below the thumb). Also, after 15 to 20 minutes, check that the thumb is not becoming numb, cool, or discolored. If it is, remove the bindings, rub the area to get things started again, and reset the restraint more carefully.

Numbness of the thumb can take several days to resolve even if the pressure that caused it lasted only half an hour. In extreme cases, it is possible to destroy the sensitivity of the thumb permanently. Checking bindings, especially at the wrist, is a basic and vital part of being a decent Top.

The second category of danger involves the bones of the wrist. These can be dislocated or broken by blows to, for instance, the back, if the bottom is hanging from or placing a great deal of weight on the bindings at his wrists. The weight of a bottom's body sagging forward against no other support than his feet on the floor and the bindings at his wrists can be bearable and none too dangerous. Certainly, if this weight becomes unbearable (and potentially dangerous), the bottom is likely to know it and shift his weight to his whole skeleton by standing up a bit. But, when a heavy blow lands on the same bottom's back, his sagging weight *plus* the force of the blow may suddenly be a greater forward thrust than his wrists can bear. You needn't understand the complicated mathematics to see what can happen here.

Good Tops learn to watch for this sort of thing, and to correct it within the dynamic of the scene. "Stand up straight, slave, and take your whipping like a man!" The order corrects the problem without so much as suggesting there was a potential danger under examination.

Ankles and Feet

The ankles are not as susceptible to injury as the wrists, although they should never be subjected to any striking or pounding. Tendonitis is easily caused by crushing and bruising the ankles. Long periods (perhaps as brief as 45 minutes) of overly tight bondage at the ankles can leave the joint unable to control or even lift the foot for hours or days. This makes a bottom hard to recycle–who wants to abuse a damaged bottom?–which is reason enough to avoid it. But, in any case where damage that lasts for days is possible, long-term and permanent damage are also possible.

If the hands are bags of nerves, bones, and tiny muscles, so are the feet, although they are a bit tougher. It is not a good idea to attempt any torture of the tops of the feet–although any part of the foot is a good site for tickling, licking, and sniffing. Still, with nothing more than normal caution, the bottoms of a bottom's feet can be a lovely torture site. Heat tortures, flogging and beating with appropriate instruments, slapping with the open hand, tickling, chilling with ice cubes, and pricking with pins and pin wheels can all be done safely.

Skin

The skin's primary task from a medical point of view is to provide a barrier between the body and the environment. This barrier is our first line of defense against infection and the introduction of foreign elements and microscopic objects, living and dead, to the internal systems. Many leathersex scenes can break the skin, as in an intense flogging, and some are, by definition, impossible without breaking the skin, as with piercing, so it is urgently important that every player understand the risk of infection and protect against it, and that care be taken not to introduce anything to the area of broken skin unintentionally.

A tattoo, for example, is an intentional introduction of foreign material into broken skin. The dirt or rust on a piercing needle, which should have been sterilized or discarded, is an unintentional introduction of foreign material. Tattoo pigments have been developed for safety, and tattoo artists learn a great deal about sterile technique and protecting their clients (and bottoms) from infection. Dirt and rust are not safe and, even if sterile conditions are hardly possible in the playroom, a Top who cannot provide clean conditions and proper care, has no right to do anything that will or might break the skin.

Circulation

It is not generally recognized by untrained people that gravity and muscle movement are important parts of the circulatory mechanics. When a person is not allowed to move his legs, for instance, the heart is being denied the useful help ordinarily provided by the larger muscles of the legs squeezing blood vessels. These muscles—and to a lesser extent all muscles—help keep the blood moving when they are functioning normally. Sometimes cramps and numbness in the muscles are messages from the body that might be interpreted as, "hey, move a bit, give your heart a helping hand here."

Massaging restrained muscles, whether presented as massage or in the guise of touching a body unable to resist the Master's hand, can help. Even pounding and beating can be acceptable substitutes for normal muscle movement in this regard sometimes. And, it is always possible to orchestrate a bondage scene so that the circulation is not much tampered with in the first place, or so that blood movement gets periods of muscle support after periods of motionless nonsupport.

PREEXISTING MEDICAL CONDITIONS

To explain all the special play space procedures that might be needed to accommodate players with preexisting medical conditions would easily fill a separate book. Everything from contact lenses to heart problems, recent bruising to diabetes should be considered. Every leathersex player should be aware that all his medical history and predispositions, and any current medical conditions (including any medications he may be taking) arrive in the playroom with him. These things can profoundly influence what kind of play is possible, what is safe, and what is to be avoided.

In most cases, the responsibility for discovering and disclosing preexisting medical conditions is shared by the Top and the bottom.

While Tops should not feel the need–except when contemplating the most extreme scenes–to take full medical histories from bottoms, they do need to be alert to signals that may suggest there are questions to be asked. Sudden shortness of breath, an unsteady gaze, trembling, and other unusual physical manifestations can signal a problem that should be looked into, at least by asking the bottom if there is a condition he wants to mention. Tops should not try to guess whether they are seeing diabetic symptoms or blood pressure problems, nervousness or an impending seizure. The only way to know what the visual cues mean is to ask.

Of course, the Top should not have to ask. Regardless of the nature of the medical condition, if there is any reason to think it might have an effect on the action in the scene, the bottom should speak up before the action gets going.

Contact lenses, for instance, can be jarred loose, creating both the possibility of losing the lenses and, in some cases, the danger of eye injury. Also, a person wearing contact lenses sometimes discovers that he cannot wear a blindfold for long without taking the lenses out first, particularly if the blindfold touches or puts even slight pressure on the eyes. Others have no such problem.

People with blood pressure problems, or heart rhythm irregularities, and people taking medications that alter their sensations or suppress their sense of pain are especially liable to problems in the playroom. But there are no medical conditions that have to preclude any possible forms of leathersex, unless they also preclude any other physical activity.

The important issue here is that every player needs to make sure that the men he plays with *know* everything that could be relevant about him. It is at least rude, possibly life-threatening, to let your partner be surprised by a medical condition you already knew about. Further, if you are a serious player, you should tell your doctor about your SM involvement and how you play, then ask him if anything in your medical condition has a bearing on what you intend to do. Remember, you don't need his approval or permission, just the information he is paid to provide.

Karl, a serious player in my circle of SM friends in Switzerland, was very eager to explain to Tops that they could keep him in a pretty small cage, get him into suspension bondage very easily, and keep him from running away with no special problem. All they had to do, he said with a totally disarming grin, was order him to remove his artificial legs. Meantime, while wearing his prosthetic limbs, he could stand for a flogging with the best of us. Karl is a good example. Not only did he not let his preexisting conditions stop him from playing, he put the conditions to work to increase the pleasurable options for his Tops. What's more, knowing that any Top he played with would sooner or later discover his prosthetics was not really the issue. He was also allergic to silk and the oil in sheepskin, and he never failed to mention it. He was just playing fair, seeing that all the potentially meaningful information was given.

Sometimes guys with what they call "a lot of padding" present themselves as safer targets for heavy beating and flogging. If the padding is layers of heavy muscle, they're right. If it is primarily fat, on the other hand, they are not so right. Fat tissues can be damaged relatively easily, and when the fat is thick enough, a heavy blow can start bleeding far enough below the surface that it is not immediately noticeable. There is, of course, no hard-and-fast rule about striking fat tissues, but don't accept the idea that fat padding makes heavy beating safer. Retain all your usual safety precautions. In the end, the fat bottom is responsible for understanding what his fat does–it prevents the Top from being certain of the exact effects of a beating. It is also the bottom's job to deal with what his limits are and ought to be. Meantime, if you're a Top who wants to pound one or more fat-padded bottoms regularly, you can take the time for a little postscene investigation. Often, you will discover surprising degrees of bruising that appeared long after the scene–evidence of bleeding in the fat tissues. It will be up to the bottom to decide if this is an acceptable result of play or something not to be repeated.

FIRST AID

Every home should be prepared to provide all kinds of first aid. Unfortunately, few homes are so prepared. When you do leathersex, your responsibility to prepare for emergencies is multiplied ten-fold or more, even if injuries from house cleaning chores, bathing, and sports are much more likely than unintended injuries from leathersex. It is a matter of moral responsibility and not open to discussion. Preparation is imperative, but easy.

A standard first aid kit, the kind made for industry rather than home, is a good idea. It will include bandaging necessities, antiseptics, gauze or some other material able to be used as a sling for an injured arm, a tourniquet, and something odorous like smelling salts. Every player should also know CPR and other first aid techniques to help people clear the breathing passages and breathe normally.

The most likely medical emergency in a well-ordered and safe scene is fainting. People faint for all kinds of reasons, and the effect is the same whether it is brought about by fear, shock, stress, or ecstasy. The only home remedy for fainting is to get the victim lying out flat, and elevate his feet. If he doesn't come to immediately, smelling salts or ammonia might disturb him into consciousness. If he remains unconscious for more than a minute, you should be prepared to call for an ambulance to deliver him to the nearest emergency room.

In the event that someone begins to bleed, anything more than the slight bit associated with piercing or the breaks in the skin from a cat-o'-nine, you should know how to stop the bleeding, including how to use a tourniquet safely. Generally, pressure at the point of the bleeding is adequate for most wounds, and, you should never use a tourniquet if you are not sure how to do so safely. Using one ineptly can cause more damage than bleeding in many cases. Also, any bleeding at all obviously means that skin has been broken, so institute your chosen method for preventing infection. In most cases and for most people, keeping the area clean after the scene, and until the skin closes up, is adequate treatment.

Men who are going to be doing leathersex, Tops and bottoms alike, should consider taking formal training in first aid. It wouldn't be a bad idea for everyone to do so, but it makes SM players safer playmates. Besides, first aid classes generally include some pertinent information about anatomy and physiology too, which can only improve your options for playing safely.

AIDS AND OTHER STDS

Frankly, leathersex has always been safer sex than nonleather sex with regard to any and all disease transmission. Grovelling, begging, spanking, following orders, and taking an ordinary flogging transmit no germs. Neither do sterile techniques like piercing and catheterization undertaken in sterile (or even carefully clean) conditions. Nor are seemingly "dirty" practices like bootlicking, armpit nuzzling, or tongue baths significant in disease transmission.

Raunchier activities like rimming (oral-anal licking) and piss drinking are hardly specific to leathersex, but they are no more dangerous in a leather context than anywhere else, and perhaps even safer. After all, leathermen–more than most others–have been forced to think about safety, and that thinking usually includes making *informed* choices about rimming and piss as well as heavy beating, bloodletting, and tight restraints.

Leathermen know that they often deal in dangerous activities, so they are inclined to consider safety for their version of sex. That being the case, they not only started out safer than many others when the AIDS crisis brought all STDs to the fore, but they were more receptive to the possibility that changes would be required. When latigo leather restraints were replaced, 15 or so years ago, by softer leather ones and later by restraints with padding and fleece lining, it didn't take leathermen long to realize that their safety was worth the change, even if the new restraints were less "serious" looking. Leathermen, for all their vaunted conservatism and solidity, change and grow pretty easily for safety's sake.

Another element in the "standard" leathersex repertoire that makes SM safer than most sexual expression–in terms of disease–is the fact that leathermen are openly, even urgently sexual, and correspondingly willing (even overeager) to talk about sex. So, safe sex information gets around fast.

Still, it has to be admitted that, even if leathermen have been in the forefront of safer sex education and the promotion of adjustments in sexual practices, some of the things leathermen do are potential disease transmission opportunities. Nonetheless, given only ordinary precautions, secured by ordinary sobriety, consensual SM interplay can be safe sex.

Ass toys have to be thoroughly cleaned and disinfected between uses–most of them can bear a 10% bleach solution, and those that cannot should probably be one-ass toys. Whips that have drawn blood need to be cleaned with a mechanical cleanser, something like hydrogen peroxide that will float away impurities, then thoroughly air-dried, and reconditioned before they are used on a different bottom. Instruments made to be inserted into the body–needles, sounds, catheters, knife blades, scalpels, etc.–must either be single-use, disposables, or sterilized between uses. That's *sterilized*, not just cleaned and disinfected. An autoclave or pressure cooker is called for, not a chemical.

Cracked, broken, or uncleanable toys must be mended to original surface integrity or discarded to avoid harboring colonies of amoebas or potentially harmful germs. Metal toys that are meant for extended bodily contact (butt plugs, collars, etc.) have to be checked to see that they really are made of benign metals. Lead is never benign, aluminum seldom is. Some people develop metal allergies, and most people are at least slightly allergic to nickel (which is common in shiny, supposedly chrome, plating).

Obviously, condoms are absolutely essential when fucking, leather power exchange notwithstanding. Many leathermen also choose to use condoms on their ass toys, including dildos, ass eggs, and butt plugs. And it doesn't hurt to also use latex (not vinyl) gloves for manual ass play and fisting, although it is very likely that keeping clean before, during, and after the scene will be just as effective. Generally, it is accepted today that cocksucking is safe without a condom, but that, like everything in sex, is your choice. Get informed, and make your own decision.

No one can claim that piss is always safe, but it appears to be AIDS-safe. As mentioned in an earlier chapter, certain infectious organisms can survive in urine. You decide whether the risk is tolerable when balanced against the pleasures, but know what you are balancing.

Scat and rimming are certainly not disease-safe, and some guys still decide to lick unwashed asses and even eat shit. That's their choice, and we can only guess that they know (from their own medical records if nothing else) what their decision implies.

Anyone, even a heavy bottom, can set limits and demand that they be respected. One reasonable demand is that all sex be safe sex by the standards of the more restrictive partner, whether that means the Top or the bottom.

Chapter Eight

Leathersex and Spirituality

Personal ads of leathermen seeking partners, articles published in leather magazines, and conversations at leathersex parties all suggest that the past several years have been a boom time for spiritual interests and practices in leathersex circles. Men are often seeking not just a flogging, but a ritual flogging, not just an SM scene, but a ritualized scene, meaning a scene more likely to involve spiritual experience. The magazines, obviously both responding to and guiding the community they serve, are publishing pieces about transcendant experiences, the spiritual movement, and the *meaning* of leathersex in psychological and spiritual terms. And, discussions that were once about how good a man felt after a particular scene are often conducted now in the vocabulary of spiritual practice which, only a decade ago, would have raised eyebrows in most leathersex circles.

It isn't that new kinds of inner experiences have recently begun to occur in the leathersex playroom. What has changed lately is that leathermen are according one another a greater degree of freedom in the discussion of their experience. This, very likely, has to do with the relaxing of the Old Leather attitudes. (It was considered inappropriate or foolish, perhaps even ridiculous, for bottoms to speak of *enjoying* the abuse they begged for as recently as the early 1970s. And any discussion involving the word "spirit" was certainly unlikely in most circles.)

Tops have always been pretty much at ease talking about their desires, and with their very closest friends they have talked technique freely, but the Old Leather attitude toward any discussion of inner experience–particularly in terms that suggest a spiritual connection–has traditionally been, "Can it! I have no idea what you're talking about."

Bottoms also talked to bottoms even in the strictest leather circles, and what they mainly talked about in the old days was the Tops they knew. One of the inhibiting factors on bottom to bottom conversation in Old Leather was the certainty that anything said to a bottom could be repeated to a Top if demanded, meaning that even when no Tops were present a bottom was risking eventual ridicule by Tops for mentioning the unmentionable.

Throughout the 1970s there were numerous independent movements and individuals working out and exploring the spiritual possibilities in leathersex. Geoff Mains, author of the classic *Urban Aboriginals*, was a very serious student of the spiritual implications of both submission and pain-bearing. Fakir Musafar (publisher of *Body Play* magazine and presenter of workshops all over the world) was very actively pursuing the pain-related spiritual practices of traditional cultures, from the Native Americans to the Hindus of the Indian subcontinent. Purusha Larkin, author of the infamous *The Divine Androgyne*, was narrowly but very deeply focused on the self-realization and spiritual liberty he discovered in fisting and other intense ass play. Also, small circles of leatherfolk were turning to Wicca (traditional, nature-power religions), to the resurgent religions of Native Americans, to Caribbean religions involving Christianity but hardly related to the mainstream of that faith, and in larger numbers to New Age spiritual practices, often personally, even eccentrically defined.

What everyone was attempting was much the same. They wanted a framework within which to understand, to communicate, and to facilitate the repetition of spiritual experiences they had (or had heard of) in leathersex. They wanted to validate their experience, and to be able to predict it or cause it to recur. Another major force involved here was the implication that experiences as intense as the ones people had with SM–usually completely unexpectedly–could be dangerous as easily as they could be transformative in a positive sense. So, as with so much in leathersex, safety became a motive for change.

Black Leather Wings, a network of men and women involved in leathersex and related to the Radical Faeries, emerged in the late 1980s as a social forum in which people could bring their various experiences and interests, their extremely divergent backgrounds, and their hopes. At gatherings (sort of faerie versions of the bike run) and at in-town meetings, the "leather faeries," as Black Leather Wings folks are often known, have given at least a certain segment of the leathersex population a comfortable context, an accommodating intersection rather than a set of doctrines.

In recent years, presentations on the spiritual dimensions of leathersex have become very popular at NLA International's annual Living in Leather conferences, in the programs of major leather/SM organizations like GMSMA in New York, and on the schedules of businesses like San Francisco's QSM set up to provide leathersex education. The word is definitely out that, although some people continue to resist the possibility of spiritual experience in the leathersex arena, it is a genuine and acceptable interest shared by a growing segment, perhaps even a majority, of the community.

WHAT ALL THE TALK IS ABOUT

While the popular forms of the world's major religions stress various codes of behavior to the exclusion of any active, personal search for truth, there are deeper levels of even the great faiths where direct experience is valued. These include the monastic mystics in Christianity and the Dervishes in Islam for instance. Many of the saints of the Catholic Church, for example, largely excluding those beatified by the earliest traditions and those recently canonized for doing good deeds, achieved their sainthood by recording ecstatic experiences. A lot of these saints–usually living under vows of chastity–expressed their vision in sexual terms, none more heatedly perhaps than Saint Theresa of Avila.

That same *type* of experience, not to depreciate the visions of the saints, is what leathersex players sometimes encounter. Placing the body at the center of one's own attention and pushing it to levels of intensity in physical experience that are not normally encountered, we discover incredible responses and "see" remarkable things. First balancing, then pushing the mind beyond the recognition of balance and imbalance, where the dominant and submissive, active and passive, self and not-self seem to be very arbitrarily defined, we enter into a peace and a sense of wholeness not available under ordinary circumstances. There, memory and expectation, regret and hope, ability and incapacity are resolved and irrelevant.

In ecstatic states, however they are arrived at, there is an inescapable sense of personal well-being based on the vision that one is intimately related to, integrally a part of, a wholeness that is perfect. The spiritual seeker–leatherman or not–is seeking to do three things above all else: He wants to experience this ecstatic condition often; he wants to grasp the meaning of the "higher" state in terms of his ordinary life; and he wants to improve himself by becoming continually more like the "perfect" self he experiences in ecstasy. Some men, calling themselves by various names but most properly shamans, also seek to teach others to achieve these visions. In leathersex circles this is often done by facilitating SM scenes, usually by Topping in highly ritualized scenes.

Some people believe that to pursue spiritual experience in SM is a mistake, and their position makes sense. There is always the danger that experience as intense as this might leave a person psychologically damaged if nothing else. And, in SM, there is also the danger that the scene may be allowed to go too far or too fast when physical pleasure has to take a back seat to spiritual intentions. Furthermore, there is a real danger that some men who claim to do leathersex for spiritual purposes are just attempting to sanitize their erotic propensities, leading to all kinds of confusing and unsafe dishonesty.

For safety's sake, then, it would seem that the right way to deal with the spiritual implications of leathersex is to understand what might be experienced in a way that makes the fear of it manageable, and stop there. Knowing what can be known without personal experience sets the psychological stage for being able to accept what happens when it comes, but it does not set up the dangerous compulsion to push toward anything. Doing SM for the right reason–because it is a joy–will sometimes lead to a surprising experience, and sometimes that experience will be best understood in spiritual terms. That is all.

Shamans and guides, like Fakir Musafar in Northern California and Stuart Norman in North Carolina, promise a degree of safety that may be what is called for when a man wants to do SM for the sake of the spiritual experience he may achieve. Unless a seeker also happens to be able to enjoy SM for its own physical and erotic attractions though, *and* already has some intimation of the ecstatic state, it is doubtful that even the experienced shamans can create a space in which this will actually take place.

WHY LEATHERSEX INVOKES SPIRITUAL EXPERIENCE

The twin engines of human spirituality are sex and death. In the mainstream religious businesses (the Christian churches) these are dealt with in bizarre ways. Death is the threshold between life and the hereafter, reduced to a dimensionless barrier with no discernable characteristics of its own. Sex is also managed by reduction. Anything that might be sex but is not within the prescribed procreative limits is simply taboo. End of discussion. To be able to do this, Christians must ignore the first book of the Bible in which sexual awareness and the knowledge that they would die were presented to Adam and Eve. They were suddenly on their own to accomplish whatever they might with their lives.

Sex and death, creativity and dissolution, are the most persistent themes in spiritual practice. Meditation is, for instance, a form of ego-stilling that tends toward dissolution of the known self. Tantric practice takes erotic ecstasy to the limit with the intention of evoking the orgasmic level of experience as a sustainable event. Even the Lord's Prayer involves the promise of some level of personal "dying" in the wish to have a higher will than one's own take over–*"Thy* will be done."

In intense enough leathersex scenes involving dominance and submission, the effects prayed and meditated for are acted out and realized. "Your will," the bottom is saying, "not mine. I am nothing, you are all." The "death" implied by the erasing of personal importance, the liberating effect of having no need to choose or decide, judge or prefer, carried on long enough, honestly enough, and intensely enough evokes states that are understandable only in either spiritual terms or those of the most sophisticated psychology–a distinction that has more to do with modern linguistic history than anything else.

Pain scenes that reach a certain level also connect us to our mortality. In fact, one way of understanding pain is simply that it is a warning signal–this way lies the danger of dying, retreat or resist.

Like submission, the intentional bearing of stimulation that the body has been trained to avoid becomes a sort of handshake with the outer edge of death, proof that although death is the threshold of eternity or oblivion, there is also an inner territory there, not just an immeasurably fine line.

The role of the erotic in all of this is somewhat harder to pin down in genuinely comprehensible words, but it is important. Put simply, when a man approaches death, whether the momentary death of his ego or physical extinction, he is likely to be overcome by fear. When he approaches the same psychological and spiritual reality of death, with its physical implications as well, in a state of sexual arousal, he is in the presence of the creative force, the balancing and mitigating energy of becoming.

The peak of spiritual experience, in one way of describing it, is to be in a state where the creation and destruction of everything existing are seen as constant. Not merely cancelling one another out, but working in such a way as to force what is created to be always an improvement on what was destroyed so that destruction is one of the powers driving more permanent and perfect creation. At its most mundane level, this understanding is expressed (however blindly) by parents who want to see their children have a better life than they have had. At a much higher level, in the mystical visions of the saints, it is the building of New Jerusalem, the making of new heavens and a new earth. And, in the experience of a leatherman, it is the sense in which what happens to him in the dungeon results in spiritual growth.

Leathersex works, even for its simplest reasons and most trivial pleasures, with creation and destruction, sexual energy and the possibility of one sort of death or another. Without both forces, the scene is unlikely to achieve anything satisfactory for either party. Still, ecstatic states worthy of description in spiritual terms are rare. They happen when the scene is sufficiently intense, when time enough is spent on the more ordinary conditions of creating a good scene, and when, to put it bluntly, the men involved are expressing enough love to create an environment where the bottom will feel completely safe "letting go," embracing the *destruction* side of the power exchange.

If spiritual ecstasy is rare for leathersex bottoms, it is many times more rare for Tops. Nonetheless, it is accessible. A Top who is satisfying no urge but his own need to dominate another man or a sadist who is beating a masochist with his own joy in mind to the exclusion of giving pleasure to the bottom will never experience what is sometimes called "the SM orgasm" or any cathartic, trans-formative, and visionary condition which can be called spiritual. The same is true of a man who is so deeply engaged in the process of pleasing the bottom that he is working at it without recognizing his own needs at all. The breakdown of the power exchange for what-ever reason cripples the scene.

On the other hand, a Top who is intent on expressing his love for the bottom, who dominates as much in response to the bottom's submission as in answer to his own needs, who stimulates for his own pleasure without losing track of the pleasure he is also giving, can be swept up in the energy changes the bottom is experiencing in such a way that he too snaps into an ecstatic state. Even if the two players are strangers, it is possible for the leathersex to be love-mak-ing, and for the power exchange to be well enough grounded in their mutual interest in pleasing one another for the distinction between the Top and the bottom as such to blur, tacitly giving control of the scene to the force they create by working together.

The effect of working together for the satisfaction of both men in a scene is that, to use a description coined by Fakir Musafar, the Top who would ordinarily have sent the bottom on a journey is now riding with him on his journey. Fakir usually speaks of this in terms of the Top either launching a boat that will take the bottom "else-where," or getting in the boat with him and rowing it, meaning he arrives at the destination with the bottom. The image captures the essence of the options perfectly, and the Native Americans even had a word for the shamanic position of the rower, one which Fakir uses: Kaseeka, meaning an experienced person who works at help-ing others acquire the experience he has.

WHAT IT ALL MEANS

It would be easy to come to the conclusion that leathermen are probably better people because of the sexual and potentially spiritual experience they have. In one way, that conclusion would be accurate. That is, the men who desire leathersex are better people if they do it than if they make a point of not doing what they want. After all, those desires are born in the complex of mind, emotion, body, and spirit that is a man's self. Getting what he honestly feels a need for is very unlikely to be bad for anyone.

On the other hand, what is true of leathersex is true of other things a man can do. Anything at all, done with the appropriate intensity and focus, can become a spiritual discipline or lead to spiritual insight. The Japanese developed the art of serving tea as a spiritual practice. Karma Yoga, by definition, is the performance of the requirements of ordinary life in such a way that sweeping, cooking, or running errands can lead to insight or even Nirvana. So, if leathermen run a higher risk of experiencing spiritual ecstasy, it is only that their pleasure-driven desire happens to pull them in a direction where achieving extremely intense experience is more likely than it is, say, for a person serving tea.

The spiritual existence of human beings is inevitable. Put another way, in a phrase that is sometimes heard in leathersex circles, we are not human beings seeking spiritual experiences, but we are spiritual beings having a human experience. Whatever the underlying truths may be, this conception of what it means to be human is useful for grasping and ordering experiences that are otherwise incomprehensible.

If we are spiritual at all, then we are spiritual all the time. Just as we continue to exist physically when our center of attention is mental, and we continue to exist emotionally when our attention is on physical activity, we continue to exist spiritually when we think, feel, or do anything. All our various parts, visible and invisible, are constantly being reshaped and influenced by all our other various parts. So, it is impossible to think that anything we do is not related to everything we are. Our experience in every realm–thought, emotion, action, and spirit–both depends upon our previous experience in all realms and changes the possibilities for future experience in all areas.

Sex is no exception. In fact, because mental, emotional, and physical (not to mention spiritual) energies are tightly interwoven in sex, it is a kind of experience that contributes powerfully to the changing and growing we do constantly. This is all the more true with leather-sex, involving as it does more extreme experiences of the body, more complex mental choices, and more intense emotions than most other sexual encounters.

Appendix A

Where Did Leathermen Come From?

If it were possible to write a comprehensive history of sadomasochism, it would have to begin in the undeciphered pictograms of our cave-dwelling ancestors. This is entirely logical since, in point of fact, there is no sexuality more deeply rooted in–even biologically dependent upon–the giving and bearing of threatening and/or painful stimulation than that of the older (and lower?) animals.

The history of what we recognize as the leather community today is not so hard to trace, nor is it at all ancient. At the risk of being considered politically preposterous, I would venture to say that the heterosexual, lesbian, and more recent "queer" and faerie leather communities descend from the gay male leather traditions in the way that North American culture derives from Western European traditions. It is not that there haven't been other influences, but that there has been one dominant model, one basic reality against which the rest are measured and of which, to varying degrees, the newer communities imagine that they are new *parts* or *improvements*.

That basic subcultural reality, the gay men's leather community, has not been carefully documented, but it has left a powerfully visible trail, a traceable record of itself right back to its beginnings. Fortunately, Gayle Rubin is preparing a manuscript (to be published as *The Valley of the Kings*) that will document and clarify that history. What is presented here is not the history itself, nor even an outline of the history. It is barely a cocktail-party answer to the question "Where did leathermen come from?"

THE HISTORY

The earliest recognizable trace of the subculture of gay leathemen is in the period immediately after World War II. During the war, many men (my father among them) had found comfort in a number of things that they were ill-equipped to live without when they came home. The strict orderliness of rank and respect, the intimate camaraderie of men sharing life-threatening stress, the comfortable grasp of who was who discerned by what a man wore, and the explosive man-to-man sexuality that evolved in the absence of women who were "safe" to hump with.

Obviously, most men and women returning from the war found ways to cope with the Ward and June Cleaver-style context of life on the home front, but not all. Some, instead, kept the sexual secrets and the military context alive. They sought out the at-home counterpart of the erotic training they had gotten in the trenches. They found it in the districts of shipping wharves and loading docks of New York, San Francisco, New Orleans, and Los Angeles where there were bars and outdoor gathering places, to be approached by strangers, as the rumors went, "at your own risk."

The risks were great. Many a veteran must have found himself battered beyond his consent, but well enough served *sexually* to return—even every weekend—to the "at your own risk" sites. Early gay guides are full of AYOR warnings, but the places were still listed, long years after intentionally gay bars were established in most major cities. In fact, AYOR notations seemed to remain in effect for leather bars once they came into existence, proving that the writers of guides were as mystified and frightened by the nascent leather world as anyone else.

Very gradually, it seems, gay vets and their home front appreciators and comrades began to infiltrate the gay bars and parties they could find. They brought with them the basic sensibilities and much of the form of the developing gay men's leather community. Sometimes they wore (despite risky legal situations) their rank-defining uniforms, or depended on meeting up with other guys who knew what insignia they had earned a right to wear. So uniforms and their meanings became part of the language of the community from the beginning. Sometimes they brought subordinates to the bars, giving rise to the kinds of service the community would soon define as Master and slave, and eventually see also in the Daddy-boy context. Sometimes they abused each other either in public or after leaving the public meeting place in ways that probably spawned the erotic versions of verbal abuse, humiliation, and eventually the clarified definitions of Tops and bottoms in leathersex.

From that point on, the history is fairly clear because it is a history made up of organizations and businesses, primarily of clubs and bars. Because no single circle of proto-leathermen could support a bar, they would "hang their colors" in a bar, meet there regularly, and think of the bar–which was used by any number of other people–as their "home bar." The group hanging the colors, or putting up a banner with a rendition of the club's logo, became the bar's "home club," and eventually the bar/club attracted enough business to survive without the less "macho" crowd. The club members, their admirers and fans, and people who found the potently male atmosphere interesting were unaware that they were creating a new business opportunity: the leather bar.

Leather per se may have become part of the scene primarily as an outgrowth of the motorcycle, which many American soldiers (again, my father among them) had learned to appreciate during the war in Europe. Being assigned a motorcycle meant, if nothing else, a degree of liberty and autonomy that the jeep-driving soldier didn't know. Only the highest ranking officers had the same freedom in a car, being assigned drivers along with their automobiles. And, if you were on a motorcycle, you had to wear leather protective clothing, whether at war or at home.

As the vets and their followers became a big enough market to support bars and produce bike runs and other events, they also began to be a distinct minority within the emerging gay male community. That was fine with them, they wanted nothing to do with the mincing and lisping that was so commonly expected of gay men. They became a separate and frighteningly different group. Where the rest of gay men were likely to be politically liberal, they were more often militantly (and militarily) conservative. Where other gay men were looking for acceptance within their local circles of straight friends, the leathermen expected not to be understood, and either hid themselves away or rejected their potential rejecters.

The 1960s, with the sexual revolution in tow, revolutionized the way outsiders looked at leathermen, and drew enough leathermen out of the shadows for people of all sorts to really look at the developing community of masculine gay men. And that, in a too-tight-to-be-true nutshell, is the birth of the leather community. From the 1960s through the 1980s, the change was one of increasing organization and cohesion, lessening secrecy, and improving networks over ever-increasing geography.

CHANGE?

In the 1990s, we hear a lot about the differences—usually called conflicts—between Old Leather and New Leather. The terms are used widely, but they seem to refer to different groups of people when used by different speakers in different circumstances. Maybe that doesn't really hurt anyone, but it also doesn't contribute anything to understanding across the various real and imaginary lines on the overall map of the contemporary leather/SM/fetish community.

Naturally, as a writer about leathersex, I have to think about the words leathermen use because I need to know how to use them in print. Listening carefully, I've discovered that the Old Guard is *relatively* well-defined, although there is often a lot of unwarranted emotional baggage dropped on it. Still, whether guys feel "cheated" because they missed out on its heyday, or feel threatened because they still see too much of it around, the Old Guard/Old Leather/Traditional Leather community is seen as a rigidly structured, merit and reward, mistake-punishment social structure, based on military-style ranking of initiated men. Depending where they came out, and when, and whether they value order or detest it, different men see the details of Traditional Leather very differently, but "everyone" knows it's other than his own idea of New Leather.

For some men, the introduction of their own favored nonleather material (rubber, spandex, etc.) is all the rebellion it takes to feel they have become representatives of New Leather. Others say switching roles Top to bottom, or wearing neo-primitive tattoos, or sporting body jewelry does the trick. Still others say the hallmark of New Leather is that it accommodates long-haired boys, women, lesbians, heterosexuals, or transvestites, or all of the above. Other guys argue that recognition of the spiritual elements in leathersex moves a man from Old to New, or that negotiating safe, sane scenes to which the bottom consents does it. And, most surprisingly to me, a growing number of men feel that the distinction between Old and New Leather is nothing more than a question of age.

The more I hear, the less I am convinced that there is a cohesive entity that can be called New Leather. When I took the problem to bed with me one night, puzzling over it as though the elusive answer were going to spell itself out on my bedroom ceiling, I hit on what feels like the truth: There is nothing new about New Leather. The range of people who are into radical sex and SM, people who do what is included in the broadest definition of leathersex, is not all that different in 1992 from what it was in 1964 when I first let myself be strung up and beaten. Although I didn't know about them until several years later, there were already circles of leather-clad, long-haired bikers in the sixties. They were rejecting the military standards of the group I knew, and doing it all *their* way. They liked being thought of as rebels, and–as I now know–they prided themselves on being able to take what they "dished out," meaning they were mostly switches rather than Tops and bottoms. They played in mud and grease, and mixed fringes and feathers with the heavy bike leathers they wore.

By 1972, I was aware of people who were incorporating some version of Native American rituals into what we today would call their SM play parties. By 1980, tattoo conventions, bike gatherings, and the no longer uncommon leather bars were demonstrating varying degrees of tolerance for people who, today, would identify themselves as New Leather.

Leather bars, strictly organized and enduring bike clubs, and certain kinds of social organizations had developed among the order-conscious men of the Old Guard, but the other ways of being a leatherman already existed. It's just that the style of the now-traditional leather community supported the establishment of permanent institutions, while the less-structured communities were, by definition, not participants in that structuring.

So, just as liberal politics were not invented by the hippies of the 1960s, New Leather was not invented by the rebels of the late 1980s. There is nothing new under the sun, even in leathersex. There is a real difference now, though, but it is not a new breed of leathermen. It is a new level of willingness in nearly all leather communities to merge with or accommodate leathermen who are different. As the communities draw together, their differences are pointed up and new strains of resistance are stirred in those who are uncomfortable with the potential union.

For myself, I have worked out a compromise I can live with: I want a traditional relationship at home, and I hope there will always be at least a few clubs and public meeting places where the traditions I admire will be respected. At the same time, I am ready to work at maintaining my chosen lifestyle in close, cooperative, and mutually supportive conjunction with the men *and* women of the evolving commonwealth of leather nations. I have no fear that my leather "homeland" will dissolve as it alternately stands apart from its neighbors for privacy and pleasure, and links up with all the other styles and varieties of leathersexuality for social and political purposes.

In other words, my life can go on as it does, but with a broader and ever-widening range of potential friends, playmates, and coworkers.

The changes we are seeing in the overall leather community are not only inevitable, then. They are also essential to the strength of all leather/SM/fetish communities. They need not threaten either the traditional leathermen (who have a lot to offer) nor the "rebels" of all stripes (who also have important contributions to make).

The future of all leatherfolk depends on the outcome, one battle at a time, of the war on sexual minorities being waged by conservative governments and churches. The only hope we have is to find and rely on what we all have in common as a basis for standing up together against our enemies.

Appendix B

Selected Readings

Baldwin, Guy. 1993. *Ties That Bind*. Los Angeles, CA: Daedelus Press.

Bannon, Race. 1992. *Learning the Ropes*. Los Angeles, CA: Daedelus Press.

Califia, Pat (ed.). 1988. *The Lesbian S/M Safety Manual*. Boston, MA: Alyson/Lace Publications.

_____. 1992. *The Sexpert: Selected Columns from Advocate Men*. New York, NY: Masquerade Books.

Cowan, Lyn. 1982. *Masochism: A Jungian View*. Dallas, TX: Spring Publications.

Greene, Gerald, and Carol Greene. 1974. *S-M: The Last Taboo*. New York, NY: Grove Press.

Herrman, Bert. 1991. *Trust: The Hand Book*. San Francisco, CA: Alamo Square Press.

Jackson, Master. 1992. *Sir! More Sir!*. San Francisco, CA: Leyland Publications.

Mains, Geoff. 1984. *Urban Aboriginals: A Celebration of Leathersexuality*. San Francisco, CA: Gay Sunshine Press.

Purusha (aka Peter Larkin or Purusha Larkin). 1981. *The Divine Androgyne*. San Diego, CA: Sanctuary Publications.

Ricardo, Jack. 1991. *Leathermen Speak Out*. San Francisco, CA: Leyland Publications.

Samois. 1981. *Coming To Power: Writings and Graphics on Lesbian S/M*. Boston, MA: Alyson Publications.

Thompson, Mark (ed.). 1991. *Leatherfolk: Radical Sex, People, Politics, and Practices*. Boston, MA: Alyson Publications.

Townsend, Larry. 1972, 1974, 1977. *The Leatherman's Handbook*. San Francisco, CA: Le Salon.

_____ . 1983. *The Leatherman's Handbook II.* New York, NY: Modernismo Publications.

Weinberg, Thomas, and G. W. Levi Kamel. 1983. *S and M: Studies in Sadomasochism.* Buffalo, NY: Prometheus Books.

Wiseman, Jay J. 1992. *SM 101.* San Francisco, CA: Jay J. Wiseman.

Index

Bathhouses
  SM-negative, 7
  unsafe for gang-bang fantasies,
    55-56
Batons. *See* rods and canes
Beards, as fetish, 120-122 *passim*
Bearing pain as processing method,
    112-113
Behaviors expected, 19-20
Belly, anatomy, 170
Belts
  basic, 23
  as safety measure, 169-170
  as toy, 85
Beneficial SM, 125-126
Bike clubs
  runs, 28-29
  some SM-negative, 6,7
Bikers in 1960s, 195
Black leather
  clothing. *See* clothing
  fetish
    and no SM, 20,25
    reasons for, 127
  historical shifting of stigma,
    158
  importance in scene, 20
  WWII motorcycle influence, 193
Black Leather Wings, 182-183
Bladder, full, 46
Bleeding
  in fat tissues, 176
  first aid, 177
  safety during abrasion, 88
Blindfolds
  in abrasion, 88
  and contact lense wearers, 175
  group sex, enhancing fantasy of
    anonymity in, 55
Blood pressure problems, 175
Bluffing. *See* honesty
Blurred distinction in power
    exchange creating ecstasy,
    183-184,187
Body language, 17

Body Play magazine (Musafar, ed.),
    182
Body stretching, 89
Bolt-cutters, 61, 62
Bondage, 59-65
  bags, 65
  cages, 64-65
  chain and steel, safety of
    bolt cutters, 62
    handcuff use, 63-64
    locks and keys, 62
    panic snaps, 63
    size considerations, 63
    tissue damage, 63
  cock and ball, 93
  elements of scenes, 61
  enjoyment of, 59-60
  feet, 94
  leather and specialty, 64
  mummification, 65
  nipple, 93
  in piercing scenes, 104, 106
  power exchange and, 59-61
  rope
    fancy knot myth, 61
    fantasies involving, 61-62
    safety in, 61, 62
  safety, 61-64
    ankles and feet, 173
    circulation needs, 174
    wrists and hands, 172
Boots
  acceptable, 23
  as fetish, 23, 118
Bottom
  asking for it, 124
  at 1960s play party, 136-138
  collar wearing, 21-22
  correcting power exchange,
    37-38
  definition of, 31-33
  dominant personality of, 38-40
  focus of, overly on self or Top,
    34-35,119-120
  joy of bondage, 60-61

Also available from Daedalus Publishing Company

www.daedaluspublishing.com

Spirit + Flesh
Fakir Musafar's Photo Book

After 50 years photographing Fakir Musafar's own body and the play of others, here is a deluxe retrospective collection of amazing images you'll find nowhere else... 296 oversize pages, three pounds worth! This book is a "must have" for all serious body modifiers, tattoo and piercing studios. **$50.00**

Urban Aboriginals
A Celebration of Leathersexuality – 20th Anniversary Edition

As relevant today as when it was written 20 years ago, author Geoff Mains takes an intimate view of the gay male leather community. Explore the spiritual, sexual, emotional, cultural and physiological aspects that make this - "scene" one of the most prominent yet misunderstood subcultures in our society. **$15.95**

Carried Away
An s/M Romance

In david stein's first novel, steamy Leathersex is only the beginning when a cocky, jaded bottom and a once-burned Master come together for some no-strings bondage and s/M. Once the scene is over, a deeper hunger unexpectedly awakens, and they begin playing for much higher stakes. **$19.95**

Ties That Bind
The SM/Leather/Fetish Erotic Style
Issues, Commentaries and Advice

The early writings of well-known psychotherapist and respected member of the leather community Guy Baldwin have been compiled to create this SM classic. **$16.95**

SlaveCraft
Roadmaps for Erotic Servitude Principles, Skills and Tools

Guy Baldwin, author of *Ties That Bind*, joins forces with a grateful slave to produce this gripping and personal account on the subject of consensual slavery. **$15.95**

The Master's Manual
A Handbook of Erotic Dominance

In this book, author Jack Rinella examines various aspects of erotic dominance, including s/M, safety, sex, erotic power, techniques and more. The author speaks in a clear, frank, and nonjudgmental way to anyone with an interest in the erotic Dominant/submissive dynamic. **$15.95**

The Compleat Slave
Creating and Living and Erotic Dominant/submissive Lifestyle

In this highly anticipated follow up to The Master's Manual, author Jack Rinella continues his in-depth exploration of Dominant/submissive relationships. **$15.95**

Learning the Ropes
A Basic Guide to Fun S/M Lovemaking
This book, by s/M expert Race Bannon, guides the reader through the basics of safe and fun s/M. Negative myths are dispelled and replaced with the truth about the kind of s/M erotic play that so many adults enjoy. **$12.95**

My Private Life
Real Experiences of a Dominant Woman
Within these pages, the author, Mistress Nan, allows the reader a brief glimpse into the true private life of an erotically dominant woman. Each scene is vividly detailed and reads like the finest erotica, but knowing that these scenes really occurred as written adds to the sexual excitement they elicit. **$14.95**

Consensual Sadomasochism
How to Talk About It and How to Do It Safely
Authors William A. Henkin, Ph. D. and Sybil Holiday, CCSSE combine their extensive professional credentials with deep personal experience in this unique examination of erotic consensual sado masochism. **$16.95**

Chainmale: 3SM
A Unique View of Leather Culture
Author Don Bastian brings his experiences to print with this fast paced account of one man's experience with his own sexuality and eventual involvement in a loving and successful three-way kink relationship. **$13.95**

Leathersex Q&A
Questions About Leathersex and the Leather Lifestyle Answered
In this interesting and informative book, author Joseph Bean answers a wide variety of questions about leathersex sexuality. Each response is written with the sensitivity and insight only someone with a vast amount of experience in this style of sexuality could provide. **$16.95**

Beneath The Skins
The New Spirit and Politics of the Kink Community
This book by Ivo Dominguez, Jr. examines the many issues facing the modern leather/SM/fetish community. This special community is coming of age, and this book helps to pave the way for all who are a part of it. **$12.95**

Leather and Latex Care
How to Keep Your Leather and Latex Looking Great
This concise book by Kelly J. Thibault gives the reader all they need to know to keep their leather and latex items in top shape. While clothing is the focus of this book, tips are also given to those using leather and latex items in their erotic play. This book is a must for anyone investing in leather or latex. **$10.95**

Between The Cracks
The Daedalus Anthology of Kinky Verse
Editor Gavin Dillard has collected the most exotic of the erotic of the poetic pantheon, from the fetishes of Edna St. Vincent Millay to the howling of Ginsberg, lest any further clues be lost *between the cracks.* **$18.95**

The Leather Contest Guide
A Handbook for Promoters, Contestants, Judges and Titleholders
International Mr. Leather and Mr. National Leather Association contest winner Guy Baldwin is the author of this truly complete guide to the leather contest. **$12.95**

Ordering Information

By phone: 323.666.2121

By via email: order@DaedalusPublishing.com

By mail:

Daedalus Publishing Company
2140 Hyperion Ave
Los Angeles, CA 90027

Payment: All major credit cards are accepted. Via *email or regular mail*, indicate type of card, card number, expiration date, name of cardholder as shown on card, and billing address of the cardholder. Also include the mailing address where you wish your order to be sent. Orders via regular mail may include payment by money order or check, but may be held until the check clears. Make checks or money orders payable to "Daedalus Publishing Company." *Do not send cash.*

Tax and shipping California residents, add 8.25% sales tax to the total price of the books your are ordering. *All* orders should include a $4.25 shipping charge for the first book, plus $1.00 for each additional book added to the total of the order.

Since many of our publications deal with sexuality issues, please include a signed statement that you are at least 21 years of age with any order. Also include such a statement with any email order.